DEATH, DISEASE,

AND LIFE AT WAR

The Civil War Letters of
Surgeon James D. Benton, 111th and 98th New
York Infantry Regiments, 1862-1865

Christopher E. Loperfido,
editor

Savas Beatie
California

Originally published in 2011 as *A Surgeon's Tale: The Civil War Letters of Surgeon James D. Benton, 111th and 98th New York Infantry Regiments, 1862-1865*

Library of Congress Cataloging-in-Publication Data

Names: Benton, James D. (James Dana), 1837-1892, author. | Loperfido, Christopher E., editor.
Title: Death, Disease, and Life at War: The Civil War Letters of Surgeon James D. Benton, 111th and 98th New York Infantry Regiments, 1862-1865 / edited by Christopher E. Loperfido.
Description: First edition. | El Dorado Hills, California: Savas Beatie, 2018. | Includes bibliographical references and index.
Identifiers: LCCN 2017018622| ISBN 9781611213591 (paperback) | ISBN 9781940669731 (ebook)
Subjects: LCSH: Benton, James D. (James Dana), 1837-1892—Correspondence. | Surgeons—New York (State)—Correspondence. | United States—History—Civil War, 1861-1865—Medical care. | Surgery, Military—United States—History—19th century. | United States—History—Civil War, 1861-1865—Personal narratives. | United States. Army. New York Infantry Regiment, 111th (1862-1865) | United States. Army. New York Infantry Regiment, 98th (1862-1865) | United States—History—Civil War, 1861-1865—Regimental histories. | New York (State)—History—Civil War, 1861-1865—Regimental histories.
Classification: LCC E621 .B553 2017 | DDC 973.7/75—dc23
LC record available at https://lccn.loc.gov/2017018622

Second Edition, First Printing

Savas Beatie LLC
989 Governor Drive, Suite 102
El Dorado Hills, CA 95762
Phone: 916-941-6896
(web) www.savasbeatie.com
(E-mail) sales@savasbeatie.com

Our titles are available at special discounts for bulk purchases. For more details, contact us us at sales@savasbeatie.com.

Proudly printed in the United States of America.

In memory of my friend Gregory A. Coco

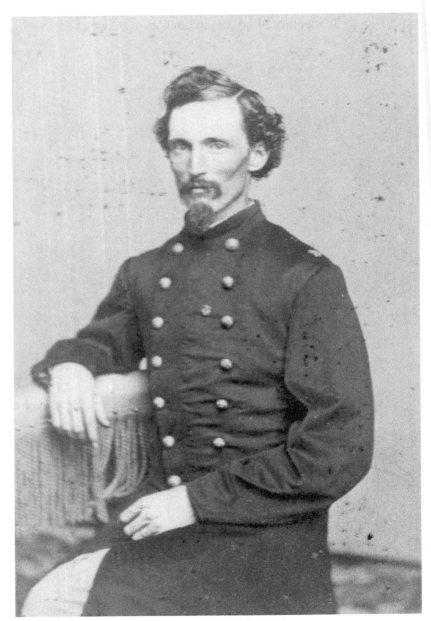

Dr. James Dana Benton

Benton Family

Table of Contents

Preface

On a crisp summer morning in August of 2008 I was looking through military folders in the Old Brutus Historical Society in my hometown of Weedsport, New York. My goal was to find letters or reports from soldiers who fought with the 111th New York Infantry, a regiment formed in 1862 from men in Cayuga and Wayne counties.

I scanned my way through the thick folders unable to find much of interest until I came across a stack of papers clipped together at the bottom of one of the folders. The papers turned out to be a series of transcribed letters written by James Dana Benton, an assistant surgeon with the 111th NY. I had read untold accounts by Union and Confederate soldiers, but had never come across a large collection of letters penned by a surgeon. The more I read, the more interested I became. The majority of the letters were filled with details about the regiment's movements, general engagements, and everyday camp life from August of 1862 until well after the end of the war in 1865. Of special interest were Benton's observations, daily concerns, and human desires, which are as witty and moving as they are intelligent and meaningful. Taken as a whole, the letters offer a relatively short but valuable memoir of what a man in his rather uncommon situation (as a regimental surgeon just behind the front lines) endured during the war. It did not take me long to determine to publish the collection.

Military Organizations

In addition to general headquarters, each army, whether Union or Confederate, was composed of infantry, artillery, cavalry, signalmen, engineers, quartermaster, commissary, and medical departments. James Benton spent his time in the service with the Union Army of the Potomac in the Eastern Theater (generally speaking, the territory between the Atlantic on the east to the Appalachian range on the west). The Army of the Potomac was the primary Union army in that region. Its opponent, the Army of Northern Virginia under Robert E. Lee, was the primary eastern Confederate army.[1]

There were three main branches in a Civil War army, consisting of infantry, artillery, and cavalry. All of these units were gathered together in an army with one to as many as eight corps, the whole commanded by a general.

INFANTRY. Generally speaking, the infantry was structured as follows:

Corps: two or three divisions commanded by a major general;

---

1 The Union followed a general policy of naming its armies after major rivers near an army's area of operations, while the Confederacy named its armies after the states or regions in a command's active area of operations.

Division: two to four brigades commanded by a brigadier or major general;

Brigade: four to six regiments commanded by a colonel or brigadier general;

Regiment: officially composed of ten companies commanded by a colonel;

Company: On paper, 100 officers and men commanded by a captain.

The word "corps" is derived from the French term *corps d'armee*. Major General George B. McClellan established the Union corps system in March of 1862. Each corps was designated with a number beginning with Roman numeral I and eventually running through XXV.[2] About midway through the war, General Joe Hooker introduced a badge or emblem system for corps, and each adopted its own, such as a red circle (I Corps), blue trefoil (II Corps), or crescent (XI Corps) to be worn by officers and enlisted men. This not only served to identify the organization, but instilled pride in the corps. The Confederates did not officially establish a corps system until November of 1862. Confederate corps were designated by number and the name of the commander.[3]

The division was the second largest unit on both sides. The Union designated divisions by badges and flags in red, white, and blue for the 1st, 2nd, and 3rd divisions, respectively. The few 4th divisions were outfitted with green badges and flags while 5th divisions were orange. The Confederates officially numbered their divisions, but over time they became known by the name of their commander.

The brigade served as the tactical fighting unit during the Civil War. Its effectiveness was largely dependent upon the ability of company and regimental commanders to teach their men complicated maneuvers and then implement them in combat.

The most important organization for the infantryman, and the one he most closely identified with, was his regiment. A regiment was composed of up to ten companies, with each 100-man company commanded by a captain

---

2 There was also a cavalry, ambulance, balloon, military telegraph, and veteran reserve corps.

3 For example, Thomas J. "Stonewall" Jackson's corps was commonly referred to as Jackson's Second Corps, or simply Jackson's Corps.

and two lieutenants. A company, especially during the early months of the war, was usually comprised of men from a single town or county. The men in each company elected their own officers. Once all ten companies were filled they would be assigned to a regiment. At full "paper" strength a regiment numbered 1,000 men and officers, but disease, absences, and casualties quickly reduced the number for both sides.

In the beginning of the war, regiments enrolled for a period of three to six months because few believed the war would last longer than that. By the summer of 1861, after the Battle of First Bull Run when it became clear the war would last much longer, the enrollment period was extended (usually to three years). Regiments were raised, organized, clothed, fed, and armed by the state until they were turned over to the Federal government. Each regiment had a flag with its regiment number, state affiliation, and was usually followed by the words "volunteer infantry." Confederate states also raised, clothed, and equipped each volunteer regiment. By 1863, many of the Confederate volunteer regiments raised in 1861 were still in service, but men called up by the draft and thus required by law to serve in the military were beginning to populate their ranks.

ARTILLERY. The long-arm of the army was usually organized by regiments and divided into companies called a battery. In the Union army, a battery consisted of more than 100 soldiers and usually six guns. Confederate batteries were smaller and usually consisted of only four guns. Batteries were assigned independently from their regiments to specific artillery brigades (as they were called in the Union, or battalions in the Confederacy), or to an army's artillery reserve. Both sides had an artillery reserve, an organization of extra batteries that would be deployed where needed during a battle.

CAVALRY. The third and final branch was the cavalry. It was organized similar to the infantry and artillery. Ten to twelve companies also called "troops" comprised one regiment. The regiment was then divided into three battalions, each usually composed of four companies. To make it easier to move in the field, a company was divided into "squadrons." Cavalry regiments were expensive to maintain because of the amount of equipment carried by each man (a carbine, saber, pistol, belt set, saddle, blanket, comb, feed, water bucket, horse equipment, and medical supplies), and the fact that each required a horse. If a horse was killed or injured, the cavalryman was relegated to foot service until a new horse could be obtained. (Most

Confederate cavalrymen were responsible for providing their own horses, many of which were brought from home).

The infantry, artillery, and cavalry units comprised an army, together with supporting organizations including quartermaster, engineer, and signal units. When the armies moved, miles of wagons loaded with food, ammunition, and medical supplies followed in their wake.

Introduction

The American Civil War was unlike any war in American history. Eleven states seceded from the United States to form their own government known as the Confederate States of America. All told, more than three million men from the North and South took up arms to fight for their respective causes. The unprecedented violence of battles like Antietam, Gettysburg, Chickamauga, and Franklin stunned everyone. By the time the guns fell silent four years later, more than 600,000 men were dead. Commonly accepted mortality figures included 360,222 from the North and 258,000 from the South. Recent research pegs that number as high as 750,000.[4] Almost as many Americans expired in captivity (North and South combined) as were killed during the Vietnam War. Hundreds of thousands died of disease. Many of the more seriously wounded survived, only to die from their wounds after the war.

Tens of thousands of books and articles have been written about this war. The vast majority study the bloody battles, the history of regiments, battle tactics, and famous military leaders like Robert E. Lee, Stonewall Jackson, Nathan Bedford Forrest, Ulysses S. Grant, William T. Sherman,

---

4 Demographic historian David Hacker from Binghamton University in New York believes that the actual death toll was more than 20 percent higher (750,000), a figure many historians and scholars are now accepting. www.nytimes.com/2012/04/03/science/ civil-war-toll-up-by-20-percent-in-new-estimate.html.

and George Thomas. Significantly fewer focus tighter to study the individuals who served in that long bloody war.

Historians prize firsthand accounts for their historical value, but the number of published primary sources account for just a small percentage of the works published on the Civil War. Many soldiers from both sides kept diaries, wrote letters home to friends and family, or gave accounts for publication in local newspapers. These letters often provide excellent insight into what the war was really like for the men who experienced it firsthand. Unfortunately, the vast majority of these documents have not survived the ravages of time. Many remain tucked away in a dusty trunk or rest unread and forgotten in a museum or some other repository.

Only a small portion of the published and unpublished letters and diaries span a significant length of time, and rarer still are accounts from the pen of men who served in the medical corps.

The letters of James D. Benton are a wonderful resource for historians and scholars of the war to gain a better understanding of what daily life was like for someone in the medical field.

Prior to the onset of the Civil War, the United States Army consisted of just 16,000 men. The medical staff was comprised of the Surgeon General, 30 surgeons, and 83 assistant surgeons. After the war began in April of 1861, three surgeons and 21 assistant surgeons left to join the Confederacy, and three assistant surgeons were dropped for being disloyal, leaving the United States medical force at a dismal 86 men. By the end of hostilities in 1865, nearly 12,000 surgeons or assistant surgeons had served with the Union army. The budget for the medical department in 1860 was $90,000. Once the war began, however, the number of diseased and injured soldiers quickly increased, and by 1863 the budget had ballooned to $11,594,000. By war's end the total medical expenditure was a staggering $47,400,000.

The man responsible for transforming the unorganized and poorly supplied Union medical department into a cohesive and efficient system was Dr. Jonathan Letterman, who was appointed medical director of the Army of the Potomac on June 19, 1862. After the failed Seven Days' Battles that ended in early July, medical supplies had been nearly exhausted and thousands of sick and wounded were left to suffer due to poor medical care and lack of medicine. Dr. Letterman recognized the need to have an organized ambulance corps and evacuation system, as well as a system of hospitals for treating the wounded. His innovations and improvements, which continued throughout the war, would save thousands of lives.

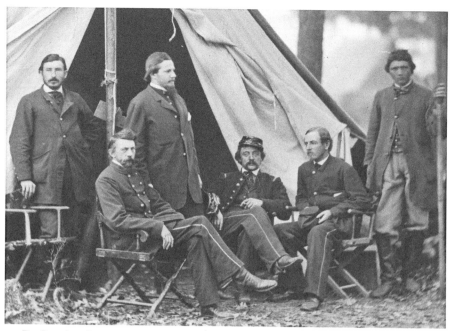

Dr. Jonathan Letterman, medical director of the Army of the Potomac and staff. *LOC*

At the beginning of the war, the initial request for 75,000 volunteers included the proviso that the regiments furnish their own surgeons. In May of 1861, an additional 40 regiments were raised, each of which was required to have one assistant surgeon commissioned by the governor of the state after an examination. Soon thereafter, the requirement was changed to include one surgeon and one assistant surgeon. After the bloody battles of 1862, particularly Second Bull Run, the army recognized that two medical officers per regiment were simply not enough, and the number was increased to three. It was typical practice to have the colonel of the regiment make the appointment and secure confirmation from a medical board. Each state differed in their selecting methods and the competence of the appointed surgeons varied; some were not even doctors. A careful examination of the medical situation was conducted by Frederick Law Olmsted of the U.S. Sanitary Commission, who reported that about seven-eighths of the appointees had been deemed inadequate, and about the same proportion had passed some type of examination.

Each man entering the medical corps was given a rank based on his level of expertise. A surgeon, for example, was given the rank of major, while an

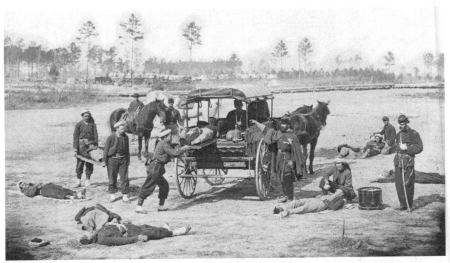

Union Zouaves demonstrating the removal of wounded soldiers from the field. *LOC*

assistant surgeon was given the rank of captain or first lieutenant. In addition to the surgeons, each regiment had a hospital steward. This enlisted man was equal in rank to a sergeant and reported to the regimental commander, not directly to the doctor.

During periods of inactivity, it was the assistant surgeon's job to conduct sick call each day, which was usually held in the morning. Every soldier who felt ill lined up to be examined. The assistant surgeon listened to the

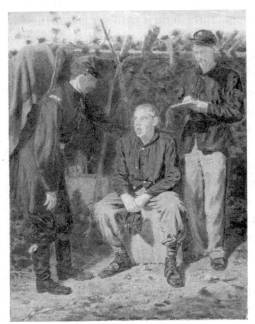

"Playing Old Soldier" by Homer Winslow. A soldier is examined at sick call by an assistant surgeon on the left, while an orderly on the right records the doctor's diagnosis for the regimental report. The term "old soldier" refers to a soldier who faked symptoms in order to avoid work or combat.

Ellen Kelleran Gardner Fund,
Museum of Fine Arts, Boston

soldier's complaints and performed a brief examination. The most common symptoms included headache, joint pain, constipation, and loose bowels. Soldiers who suffered from significant chronic disabilities were medically discharged from the army. If an illness interfered with a man's ability to carry out his usual military duties, treatment was undertaken and he was assigned to limited duty. Any illness was recorded by the hospital steward and forwarded to the next highest physician, who was usually the brigade surgeon.

Assistant surgeons faced a higher level of danger than did surgeons, who were usually stationed in field hospitals well back from the front lines. Assistant surgeons remained in close proximity to their units (which were usually on or near the front line) during battle. The assistant surgeon was the one who established an "advance" or dressing line situated behind the firing line, where the doctor could examine the wounded. Ideally, this location would be set up in a gully or depression to avoid flying lead and iron or near an area protected by trees. Because battles were not static affairs, a hospital well behind the front lines could suddenly find itself in the middle of the action.

Early in the war, surgeons often arrived in the army with a medical bag from home containing his personal surgical tools such as a catlin (a long, thin double-bladed knife), artery forceps, bone forceps, scalpel, scissors, and butted probes. The hospital steward was responsible for a knapsack containing medicines and equipment provided by the government. A typical regimental knapsack contained both chloroform and ether for use as anesthetics, lint, bandages, tourniquets, sponges, morphine, opium pills, whiskey, and brandy. In addition to the assistant surgeon and hospital steward, the dressing line included stretcher bearers, a position that required great courage. These men left the protection of the trees or depression to move out into the open and retrieve the wounded. If a soldier was unable to walk, the stretcher bearers carried him to the dressing line for medical attention.

Once a wounded solder made his way behind the firing line to the dressing line, the assistant surgeon examined his wound(s) and did everything possible to stem any bleeding. No significant surgical procedures would be undertaken unless there was an urgent need for it. Whenever possible, he would remove foreign objects from wounds (such as bits of cloth from the uniform, bullet or shell fragments, leather from belts or cartridge box straps, etc) to diminish the chance of infection. In the 1860s,

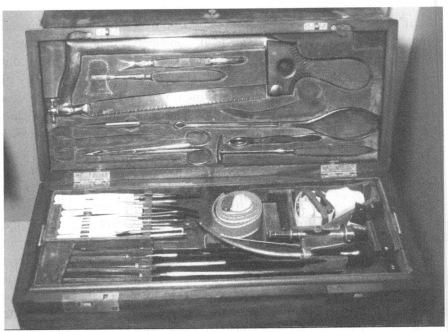

A typical surgeon's kit.
Courtesy of the National Museum of Civil War Medicine, Frederick, Maryland.

doctors had only a very limited understanding of infection. They did not understand germs or how they were carried and spread. Proper sanitary procedures were essentially nonexistent. A minor wound could easily become infected, turn septic, and kill a man. Of all the deaths during the Civil War, nearly two-thirds were from disease. The wound would then be packed with lint, bandaged, and the soldier would be directed toward the collecting point, where a wagon would pick him up and transport him with others to a field hospital farther to the rear.

At the field hospital, a wounded soldier quickly discovered he was but one of many waiting on the ground or a pile of straw for an examination and if needed, his turn on the operating table. Field hospitals were usually situated well behind the line in a place with plentiful water. Anything that could provide a shelter from the elements worked just fine, including tents, barns, sheds, stables, houses, and churches. Because wagons were needed to haul the large number of wounded, supplies, and food, field hospitals were located by at least one serviceable road so the ambulances could quickly and easily find their way to and from the battle area.

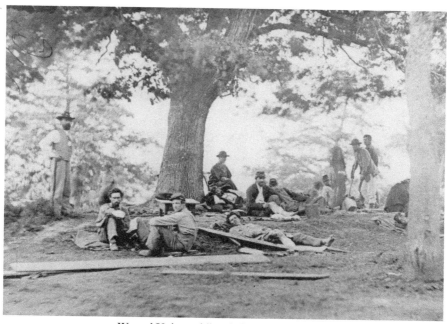

Wound Union soldiers being cared for after
the Battle of Chancellorsville in May 1863. *National Archives*

Field surgery (mostly amputations) was still in its early stages by the time the Civil War arrived. The majority of wounds treated by surgeons were to the arms and legs (because most to the body were fatal and those who suffered them were less likely to make it back to a field hospital). The procedure was usually performed on a wooden platform such as a table, or in many cases, atop doors ripped from their hinges. Shelter from inclement weather was important, so most operations took place inside a house, a barn, in an open air tent, or on some occasions, on a table outside. Amputations were often witnessed by many people, from other doctors eager to learn the procedure to the unfortunate men awaiting their turn under the knife. Maj. General Carl Schurz, who led a division in the Army of the Potomac's XI Corps, described in excellent detail the scene of an operation at Gettysburg:

> Most of the operating tables were placed in the open where the light was best, some of them partially protected against the rain by the tarpaulins or blankets stretched upon poles. There stood the surgeons, their sleeves rolled up to their elbows, their bare arms as well as their linen aprons smeared with blood, their knives not seldom held between their teeth, while they were helping a patient on or off the table or had their hands, otherwise occupied. . . . As a wounded man was lifted on the table,

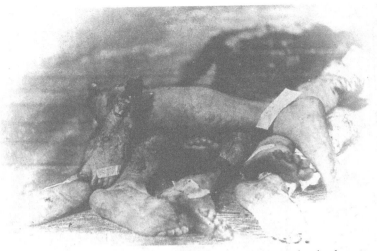

Entitled "A Morning's Work," this 1865 image was taken under the direction of Dr. Reed B. Bontecou, surgeon in charge of the Harewood US Army General Hospital in Washington, DC. *National Museum of Health and Medicine*

often shrieking with pain as the attendants handled him, the surgeon quickly examined the wound and resolved upon cutting off the injured limb. Some ether was administered and the body put in position in a moment. The surgeon snatched his knife from between his teeth. . . . wiped it rapidly once or twice across his bloodstained apron, and the cutting began. The operation accomplished, the surgeon would look around with a deep sigh, and then [shout]—"Next!"

Once on the operating table, the patient was anesthetized with ether or chloroform. Chloroform was preferred because it worked fast and was non-flammable. The liquid was dripped onto a folded cloth or sponge and held over the patient's nose and mouth until he lost consciousness. The majority of operations were for bullet wounds, which accounted for approximately 250,000 patients. Lead rounds lost their shape and expanded once they struck a man, splintering bones and tearing apart muscle tissue.

The most logical and efficient way to care for these injuries was amputation. A deep cut was made through the skin and muscle, down to the bone above the wound. The bone was sawed through with a bone saw and the severed limb tossed onto a pile of severed arms and legs, which created a gruesome sight. Once the bone was smoothed a bit, the stump was covered with skin and muscle tissue and sutured shut. The soldier was carried to

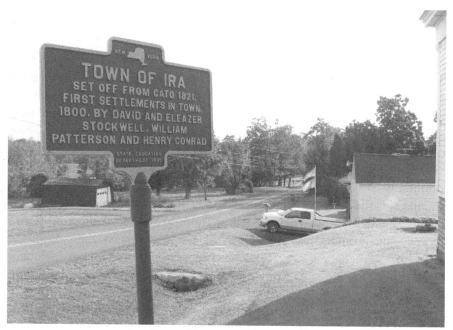

Town of Ira, present day. *Author*

another area to rest before being evacuated to the nearest general hospital, which was staffed with military doctors, nurses, and volunteers.

As an assistant surgeon, James Benton performed these and other important duties for nearly three years.

*   *   *

Allen Benton (James Dana Benton's father) was born June 9, 1792, in what is now Ira, New York, in the northeastern part of Cayuga County. He worked initially as a teacher, but had a yearning to pursue a medical career. Allen spent the next three years studying medicine under a Dr. John W. Squyers, an esteemed elderly physician in the community. In addition to medicine, Allen turned his attention to agriculture, buying a small tract of land in Ira. He added more land a few year later until he eventually owned 650 acres, one of the largest plots of land in the area. Through hard work and determination, Allen turned his land into well-cultivated and productive fields. As a successful farmer and medical doctor in a small community, Allen was one of the most prominent and influential citizens in the area and thus held in high regard. He passed away on September 12, 1877, at the age of 85.

James's mother, Deborah Willey, was born February 1, 1798, in East Haddam, Connecticut, the daughter of Abraham Willey, one of the original settlers of Cayuga County. It is unknown when she moved to Ira or when and how she met Allen, but they married on July 22, 1819. She spent her time raising five children: James, Heman, Charles, Allen, and Matilda. She passed away on August 23, 1867, at the age of 68.

James Dana Benton was born in Ira, on July 22, 1837. The small community is bounded on the north by Oswego County, on the east by Onondaga County, on the south by the town of Cato, and on the west by the town of Victory. Ira was first settled in 1800 by William Patterson, Henry Conrad, and brothers David and Eleazer Stockwell who came from the village of Whitehall, located near the Vermont border. It was officially formed on March 16, 1821 from Cato, which at the time was an enterprising village of 500 inhabitants. The new town was located on fertile country with large rolling ridges and rich in fruit and grain. The town contained a post office, one Baptist church, a school, hotel, cheese factory, two blacksmith shops, carriage shop, harness shop, milliner shop, and a tin shop. In the census of 1875, the township around Ira comprised 21,156 acres, of which 17,134 are improved. More than 3,000 acres were woodland, and another 1,000 unimproved. By the time of James's birth, Ira had a population of 2,064, four of whom were African-American.

As was common for children raised on farms, James obtained experience in several different areas of agriculture and spent much of his day helping his father with chores. James also grew up watching his father practice medicine, which is where he developed his own interest in the profession. Little is known of his late teenage years except for five letters he wrote to his parents while attending Albany Medical College in Albany, New York, where he graduated in December 1857.

After graduation, James returned home to Ira, where he met and fell in love with Cato resident Margaret A. Rich. One of eight children born to George R. Rich (a prominent Cato lawyer) and Margaret Anne Wallace, Margaret was born on October 30, 1838.[5]

---

5   Unfortunately, the only information I was able to find on Margaret's mother was that she was born to Ruloff and Maria Wood of Montgomery County, New York.

James's wife, Margaret Benton

Benton Family

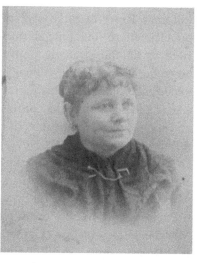

The next two years were turning points in James' life. On November 10, 1858, he and Margaret wed. The following year James put his medical degree to use by taking over as town physician from Dr. W. W. D. Parsons. On Christmas Day 1859, he and Margaret welcomed a baby girl into the world whom they named Jessie. The three enjoyed what appears to have been a comfortable and happy life until hostilities broke out on April 12, 1861. With the United States now engaged in a war with the Confederate States of America, young men everywhere were eager to help defend the Union. James would eventually sell his medical practice to physician Azariah Judson as part of his preparations for enlisting in the U.S. Army.

The war had raged on more than a year when James gave up his seemingly idyllic and peaceful life to enter the military on August 7, 1862. He left Ira for Auburn, New York, and once there enrolled in the army for a period of three years. His new regiment would be the 111th New York Volunteer Infantry. The 111th had its origins in the summer of 1862, when President Abraham Lincoln called for an additional 300,000 volunteers to aid in the war effort. On July 19, permission to raise a regiment was granted to 58-year-old Jesse Segoine, who would act as its colonel. The regiment was organized throughout the late summer and mustered into service on August 20, 1862 at Auburn. With his background in medicine, James mustered in as an assistant surgeon on August 20, 1862.

Like many regiments during the Civil War, the 111th New York would muster out at the end of war with an interesting history. At times it performed very well, but this was not always the case. Its most humiliating performance arrived just a few short weeks after it had been mustered in, earning its members the nickname "Harpers Ferry Cowards."

After a string of Southern victories in Virginia, Confederate General Robert E. Lee decided to march his victorious army north across the

Potomac River in early September 1862. The move prompted the Union government to sound the alarm and rush many of its newest recruits into the field to defend strategic points in an effort to counter the Confederate advance. Many of these men had little training and virtually no combat experience. James and his regiment were sent to help defend Harpers Ferry, a strategic position at the confluence of the Shenandoah and Potomac rivers and soon a Confederate objective for capture. With only three short weeks of military experience, the New Yorkers of the 111th, part of Col. F. G. D'Utassey's brigade suddenly found themselves deployed on Bolivar Heights, in an untenable situation against some of the finest troops in the world led by Thomas "Stonewall" Jackson.

On the afternoon of September 12, skirmishing broke out along Maryland Heights as Confederates began encircling Harpers Ferry. Hostilities resumed the following day as Jackson began closing the loop on the trapped garrison. On the afternoon of September 14, Jackson's Confederates slowly advanced south of the ferry toward Bolivar Heights. Southern artillery pounded the trapped Union soldiers, but darkness prevented a major infantry attack. The next day on September 15, the garrison's commander, Colonel Dixon Miles, fell mortally wounded from a shell burst as Jackson's foot soldiers advanced toward Bolivar Heights. General Julius White assumed command of the ferry and promptly surrendered the Union garrison.[6]

Fortunately for James and his comrades, the New Yorkers pledged they would not take up arms until properly exchanged and were quickly paroled. Once the parole process was complete, they marched about 100 miles to Annapolis, Maryland, where they arrived on September 20. On September 27, just one month after being mustered into service and their harrowing ordeal, the regiment arrived at Camp Douglas in Chicago, Illinois. The camp served as a training facility and prisoner of war camp. This is where Dr. James Benton's wartime correspondence begins.

James spent the remainder of the war in the Eastern Theater with the Army of the Potomac. He played a role in every major engagement through

---

6   Bradley Gottfried, *The Maps of Antietam: An Atlas of the Antietam (Sharpsburg) Campaign, including South Mountain, September 2–20, 1862* (Savas Beatie, 2015), 92-109. The capture of Harpers Ferry was an embarrassing and expensive loss for the Union. More than 12,000 men were captured along with 73 pieces of artillery, 13,000 small arms, and tons of equipment and clothing.

the grueling siege of Petersburg and the occupation of Richmond immediately after the fall of the city in April 1865. From a purely military standpoint, the 111th New York's most notable contribution was at Gettysburg on July 3, 1863, where the regiment performed brilliant defensive work in the bloody repulse of Pickett's Charge.

*   *   *

The original owners of James's letters, Paul and Barb Benton, informed me that they had the entire collection of letters James wrote to his parents during the war. There were 42 pieces of correspondence penned between 1862 and 1865. Oddly, there was no correspondence from November 6, 1864, to March 5, 1865, but Paul and Barb assured me that nothing was missing; for reasons unknown, James simply did not write home for nearly four months. The majority of his letters were to his father Allen, and a few to his mother Deborah. The documents themselves were all written in ink, except for a few words, completely legible and easy to read. Unfortunately, we know James wrote many letters during the war to his wife Margaret, but their whereabouts remains unknown.

Editing the letters of James has been a long, sometimes difficult, but always satisfying process. The letters are reproduced here with only minor punctuation changes and some paragraphing to enhance readability.

My hope is that you find James's honesty, raw emotion, and passion for his work as fascinating as I do. The insight contained in these letters into what life was like for surgeons during the war to help preserve our nation is simply invaluable.

Chris Loperfido

Acknowledgments

As with any book, its creation is not without the help of others. Making the letters of James D. Benton available was a direct result of Barb Benton, who worked tirelessly to transcribe them. I would also like to thank the Old Brutus Historical Society in Weedsport, New York where I found the letters that Barb had donated. The staff was more than willing to assist in my research and attempted to answer any questions I had. While the groundwork for this book was laid at the Old Brutus Historical Society, the following individuals were instrumental in my mission to complete this project. If it were not for their help and encouragement, this book would cease to exist and for that I am grateful.

First and foremost I would like to give thanks to my parents Bernie and Lynne Loperfido. From the beginning they have supported and encouraged me in whatever I chose to attempt. Thank you for your love and support.

My wife Paige, who deserves much more than a sincere thank you. Not only is she my beloved spouse, but also my best friend. She is owed more than I could ever repay.

Barb and Paul Benton, whose great, great uncle is James D. Benton. They were kind enough to meet with me, provide several pictures in this book, and answer any questions I had regarding James and his family.

I would like to express my gratitude to my former colleagues at the Gettysburg National Military Park. Gregory A. Coco, Matt Atkinson, John Heiser, and Scott Hartwig were especially instrumental in my quest to complete this book. Not only did they assist me with the many questions I had, but also aided in the location of sources for my research.

Lastly, I would like to give a sincere thank you to Theodore P. Savas of Savas Beatie, LLC, who had faith in me and my manuscript. He understood my vision for this publication and took on the many burdens and commitments which have allowed the letters of James to reach the public, including asking authors Meg Groeling and Dr. Dennis Rasbach to contribute the excellent and helpful appendices. (Thank you both.) To the rest of the Savas Beatie team who worked on this project, Sarah Keeney, marketing director, Sarah Closson, media specialst, Ian Hughes, of England who designed an outstanding cover, and Catherine Robertson for providing genealogical research, thank you all for your hard work on this book.

Once again to everyone who has aided me with this publication, thank you.

1862

James Benton's first correspondence to his father Allen was penned August 14, 1862, and is reproduced below. James was in Auburn awaiting the muster in of his regiment, which would be mustered into service on the 20th and leave for Harpers Ferry the following day. Once that was complete, the men would be outfitted and equipped by the government. Officers and surgeons would receive an allowance to purchase clothing and equipment. Doctors were expected to purchase their own surgical instruments and would be reimbursed by the government if they did not have their own kit.

* * *

Head-Quarters, Military Post
25th District
Auburn, N.Y.
August 14

Dear Pa

The officers and staff and the medical staff met last night and ordered their accoutrements from New York. The medical officers all send for the same articles. I wrote to Maggie what money I should want and what for but we have had no official meeting. The articles I will enumerate

Sword   12.00
Sash   7.00
Sword Knot   1.50
Belt   2.75
Shoulder Straps   6.50
    "   "   2.50
Spurs   1.50
Saddle & Trappings   35.00

The Colonel[1] has taken great pains to get these articles as cheap as they can be purchased. They cost about 33 1/3 percent less than the 75th Regiment[2] had to buy.

You see from this what my expenses are going to be saying nothing about my clothes which I have money to pay for now. I guess Charley[3] has got money he would lend to me. Raise the money for me and I will send my notes in for it. I send the Wormuth note. Send in an answer as soon as possible by some one coming in. I can get it sooner than by mail.

Your son
J. D. Benton

*   *   *

1   Colonel Jesse Segoine was 58 years old when he enrolled at Auburn, New York to serve three years. He was appointed colonel of the 111th New York Volunteer Infantry on July 19, 1862, and assumed command on August 15, 1862. He was discharged on January 3, 1863.

2   The 75th New York Volunteer Infantry was organized in Auburn, New York, and was composed of men from Cayuga and Seneca counties. It was mustered into service for three years on November 26, 1861, and mustered out under Colonel Robert P. York on August 31, 1865, at Savannah, Georgia. During the war the regiment lost four officers and 201 enlisted men to all causes.

3   Charley is one of James's seven siblings, two of whom died the day they were born. Charley was born April 15, 1828, and died June 21, 1907.

The 111th New York, part of Col. Frederick G. D'Utassy's brigade, found itself caught up in the Antietam Campaign, and was unfortunate enough to be stationed at Harpers Ferry in western Virginia, when it was surrounded on September 12 by converging Confederate columns led by Maj. Gen. Thomas "Stonewall" Jackson.[4]

The besieged garrison surrendered on the 15th and Dr. Benton and the men of his regiment were paroled the following day. Benton and the men of the 111th, 39th, 125th, and 126th New York regiments began the 100 mile trek to Annapolis, Maryland, where they arrived on September 20.

*   *   *

Annapolis, Maryland
Monday, Sept 22nd/62

Dear Maggie

The last letter I wrote you I directed you to write to Baltimore and instead of going there we went to Annapolis the Capitol of Maryland and we are ordered to be ready to march tomorrow and it is said we are to go to Chicago, which I think is probable as there are no accommodations for us here. Some of our officers have telegraphed to W[illia]m. H. Seward[5] to have us sent to the barracks at Auburn whether it will be so or not I can't say. I think we will go to Chicago.

4   Frederick George D'Utassy was born in Hungary in 1827, immigrated to New York City and was commissioned to lead the 39th New York Infantry. He would be court marshaled in May 1863 for illegally selling horses stolen from the army and using his rank for personal profit, serve one year in a New York City prison, and thrown out of the army. D'Utassy was found dead in a gas-filled hotel room in Delaware on May 5, 1892, perhaps by his own hand. Harpers Ferry was a strategic area at the convergence of the Shenandoah and Potomac rivers where the states of Virginia, West Virginia, and Maryland meet. John Brown launched his infamous raid there in October of 1859 in the hope of seizing its arsenal and fomenting a slave rebellion. The raid was put down by a detachment of United States Marines led by Colonel Robert E. Lee.

5   William Henry Seward was secretary of state from 1861-1869. In 1860, he had run for the presidential nomination of the Republican Party but lost to Abraham Lincoln. He served as secretary of state through Lincoln's assassination on April 14, 1865, and under President Andrew Johnson until March 1869. It was Seward's idea to purchase Alaska from Russia in March of 1867. He died on October 10, 1872, in his home in Auburn.

We are now encamped in the woods & sleep on the ground. I am tough as a bear & feel first rate (only I want to hear from home). I have had only one letter yet and you need not write until we know where we are going. We start to-morrow.

We have had a long and hard march from Harpers Ferry and [are] going a long distance out of our way. We started on Tuesday morning the 15th and arrived here last night the 21st Sept. Sleeping in the open air on the ground. At one place when we stopped I stayed at a public house and slept in a bed and I felt worse when I got up than when I went to bed. I went to our camp and laid down on the ground had a little nap and rose and felt tip top. I am not used to a bed, I can buy a piece of pork on the end of a stick and a potatoe in the ashes and make a good meal. I get along well and better than expected. I dont draw any rations as the soldiers do but I am allowed 4 rations per day equal to $1.20 per day. I live among the boys and most always eat with them.

I am not homesick but I want to see you and Jessie more than I can tell. All the letters which have been written to me could not get to me and went to Washington. Since we came to Annapolis we have sent for them and expect them all the time probably we will get them to-morrow. I never knew before how much I was attached to my family and how much I loved you and Jessie.[6]

[September] 23rd: We are waiting for orders. It is said by some that we are to go to Auburn in our own barracks. When we get settled at some place I will let you know where to write to. In two hours we will probably start for some place or other.

How I want to hear from you and Jessie. We expect our letters every moment. We sent to Washington for them several days since. When I get to some place to stay I want your and Jessies pictures & I will send you mine as soon as I can get it taken. I want to see how Jessie looks. The little bird she is such a good little girl. Tell her her Pa loves her and thinks of her often.

Good bye Maggie. I will tell you when to write when we get settled for good. Goodbye again.

Yours as ever
J. D. Benton

---

6 James's and Margaret's daughter Jessie was born December 25, 1859, and died December 5, 1942.

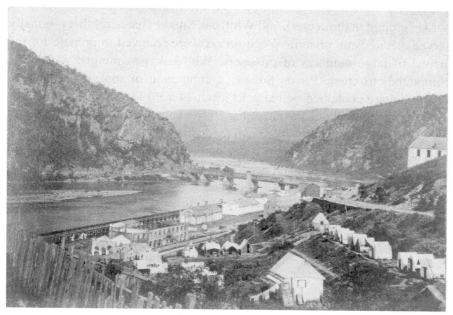

A view of Harpers Ferry. *National Archives*

---

*   *   *

Following a brief stop in Annapolis, the men were sent on to Camp Douglas in Chicago by boat and train, where they arrived around September 27. The men would remain at the camp until November 1862 and is where Benton wrote the following six letters.

Camp Douglas was originally implemented as a rendezvous point to train and house regiments established in the Chicago area at the beginning of the Civil War. The camp was established on the south side of the city on grounds originally occupied by the 7th Annual Fair of the United States Agricultural Society held in 1859. It was named in honor of Illinois statesman Stephen A. Douglas, whose residence was nearby; part of the camp sat on some of the Douglas property.

The roughly 60-acre camp was divided by interior partitions to create compounds of differing sizes. Each compound was named according to its purpose. Dr. Benton would likely have been stationed at Hospital Square, which contained ten acres and served as its name implied. Other compounds included Garrison Square (which contained twenty acres and was lined on all sides by the quarters of the officers and men and had a flat and level parade ground in the center), and Whiteoak Square (ten acres that originally served as the camp prison). When orders were received to prepare for the arrival of large numbers of prisoners, Whiteoak was merged with other compounds to create Prison Square, a compound of some twenty acres. Prison Square contained 64 barracks, each 24 x 90 feet. Some 20 feet was used for the kitchen and the remaining 70 feet contained tiers of bunks along the walls. The entire capacity was intended to be capped at 6,000 men, or roughly 95 men to a barrack, but as the number of Rebel prisoners increased, each barrack was jammed and eventually held an average of 189 men.[7]

*   *   *

Camp Douglas
Chicago, Ill.
Oct. 4, 1862

Dear Father,

I know you are anxious to hear from me, as I have not written to you in some time. I have to get along with writing but few letters as possible.

We have finally landed in the city of Chicago or near it, which you probably have learned before this. We are all well and beginning to get rested from our long journey.

I wish I could give you a long description of the capture of 8000 prisoners at Harpers Ferry. I am sorry to say I lost my saddle and bridle and I come within a hairs breadth. Peter Megrand takes care of him for me and as he was running around on the flat below Bolivar Heights he called him and he ran up to him in that way he was saved. I picked up a secesh saddle all torn to pieces and have used it until now I wish I could preserve it as a curiosity. I received a letter from Richardson to-day with a strong invitation to come to see him as I am so near only a few hours ride I enclose his letter. I should like to go very much. We have got no pay yet and we are all short of money that is

---

7   The people of Chicago were curious about the prisoners. Shortly after the camp opened, entrepreneurs developed a way to exploit the misfortunes of the prisoners. An observatory was erected just outside the prison gates. For the price of ten cents, a spectator could ascend the platform and with the aid of furnished spy or field glasses, gaze down upon the men.

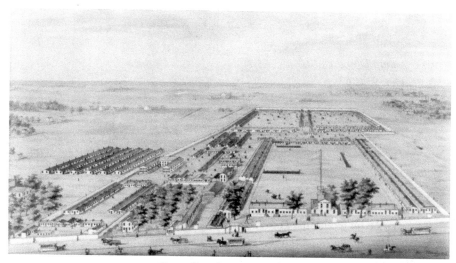

Camp Douglas. *Harper's Weekly*

the only reason. Uncle Sam owes me about two hundred and sixty dollars now and I would thank him to pay up. We are getting our old letters, which were written to us at Harpers Ferry. I received one from Maggie to-day dated Sept. 4 that is rather old you know but they are a great deal of comfort.

We have had some pretty rough times since we started more so than many regiments of our age. It is not patriotism that has made me take this course but I wanted to make money for my family. If it had been patriotism I should have been sick of it long since but as it is not my plunk is good. I am of the opinion that we will winter here but we know nothing about it. We may leave in a week but from appearances I think we are to stay.

Camp Douglas is not as perhaps you may have imagined a delightful spot. It is on pararie ground and is a muddy nasty lousy ratty hole. The guards shoot lots of rats every night. But I must close I will try to write more of Camp Douglas in my next.

Write soon & believe me

Your affectionate son
J. D. Benton

* * *

Camp Douglas, Ill.
Oct. 9, 1862

Dear Father,

I received your very welcome letter last night and proceed this morning to reply to it and I will try to answer the questions as they occur.

You advise me to go down to see Richardson. I have been trying for 4 or 5 days to procure a leave of absence and even have been sick, still I cant get it. Since I cant get it I am better.

We probably shall stay here most of the winter and if we do so I shall hope to go and see him. [I] am glad to hear that you are all in good health at home. About my learning something more about war I mean that if I should start again I would do different in many respects. I would not pay $10.00 for a bed to take with me. I would not give $35.00 for a saddle & when I can & will buy a better one for $10 or $15. I would not take a trunk filled with clothes & I would not wear a $20.00 coat and $7.00 pants. In fact I would not do a great many things that I did do. If we leave here I shall send my trunk home again. I want only what I can carry on my horse strapped behind my saddle. My horse does well and is in good condition. I would not trade with the Col[onel] for $50.00 to boot there is more difference than that in their real value for my horse knows more than any horse I ever saw.

The other surgeons of our Reg[imen]t. Dr. [William] Vosburgh[8] is in the hospital at Harpers Ferry but will probably join the Regt. soon. Dr. [Stuart] Hopkins[9] is here and I am now engaged in the office of the surgeon of this post Dr. McVickar. He has control of all the hospitals & of this post and is the medical director of the whole forces here. I am employed in his office in prescribing and as an assistant to him and for the time being am detached

8   Dr. William Vosburgh was a surgeon with the 111th New York Volunteer Regiment. At the age of 36 he enrolled at Auburn, New York to serve three years and was mustered in as a surgeon on July 25, 1862. He was mustered out with the 111th on June 4, 1865 near Alexandria, Virginia.

9   Dr. Stuart Hopkins was an assistant surgeon with the 111th New York Volunteer Regiment. He enlisted September 9, 1862 and was promoted to surgeon of the 4th Delaware Volunteers on February 6, 1863.

from our Regt. or at least as long as he wants my assistance. It is an honorable position. Dr. Hopkins is not a man after my style at all but we used to get along well enough. Dr. Vosburgh is a gentleman and all hope he will soon be with us again.

We have some wounds to dress here and we had many at Harpers Ferry. The wounds were temporarily dressed on the field and operations performed at the hospital. The first case we had was a man who had his leg torn off by a piece of shell. We amputated his leg in the upper part of the thigh but the shock to the system was so great that he died in a short time. The effects of pieces of shells are dreadful and few recover from wounds of any great extent made by them. Col. Miles had the calf of his leg torn off only and it would seem that with proper treatment, a person ought to recover from such a wound but there is so much prostration and shock that they die in most every case of extensive wound. Sunday night previous to the surrender [at Harpers Ferry] I was engaged in the general hospital dressing wounds & attending to the wounded. I cant describe by letter any of the cases so as to make it anyways interesting, suffice it to say they were all bad enough.

The sickness now in camp is considerable and is chiefly diarrhoea, dysentery[10], and the various types of fever, good deal of ague here. I was much in want of the money you sent and will repay it as soon as we receive our pay. It is said that we are to be paid the first of November if so I shall draw almost $400.00, about $390.00. That will pay up pretty well and it is making money a little faster than I have been used to.

I would present my note for payment to Wermuth immediately and get the money. Camp Douglas in good dry weather is a splendid camp and in wet weather is a nasty muddy sickly hole. It is on parairie soil and is as level as a floor, and is a sandy loam. We are 4 miles from the center of the city [Chicago]. The last of the Rebels died a few days since the rest were previously sent away probably exchanged. We are obliged to keep good company and conduct ourselves like gentlemen. We cant do otherwise. Of course there are rascals in every camp but the officers are compelled to conduct themselves properly.

---

10 Dysentery was responsible for about one-quarter of all the sickness reported in the Civil War. This infection of the digestive system results in severe diarrhea. It was usually caused by unsanitary water. Symptoms include a thickened, softened condition of the mucus membrane, with pigment deposit and enlargement of the solitary follicles, and can include blood in the feces.

[I] am glad to learn that Maggie and Jessie are well. You dont know how bad I want to see them. Give my love to all.

Write soon as possible and give me all the news.

Your affectionate son
J.D. Benton

*   *   *

October 27, 1862
[Camp Douglas]

Dear Father,

It is too late for me to write you a letter of much length but I thought I would write to let you know that we are still here and things are going on as usual. I have not been able to do any duty for several days but am getting better somewhat now. I have had what old women call the "yaller janders"[11] and I am "yaller" enough now for that matter. Co[l]. Segoine arrived today at dress parade he returned the flag to the Regt. which he said he had struggled so hard to save when the truth was that Co. Dutasay had it concealed in his trunk and kept it there. Co. Segoine having nothing to do with it. He is an old fool in my private opinion.

Let me give you an instance of his foolishness. He told Frank Rich and other officers to-night that we would be exchanged in twenty days, that he knew it from good authority because said he "we will have two severe battles in a short time and probably will take enough prisoners to exchange us." Those were his words and a man must be a fool certain that would base an opinion on such a matter. The boys are as well as usual, still we have much more sickness here than at Harpers Ferry. You speak of hospital stores. I think that the box which the ladies contemplate sending had better be sent to

11 Jaundice is a disease of the liver. It is a condition characterized by a yellowish staining of the skin, mucous membranes, and body fluids with bile pigment. It is not a disease, but is regarded as a symptom with varying origins. It is of three types: obstructive, non obstructive, and infectious. Obstructive comprises about 85% of all cases. Non-obstructive is regarded to be of splenic origin, and infectious is a symptom of some condition such as phosphorus, chloroform, or arsphenamine poisoning.

some Regt. in the field as the people of Chicago supply us very well but if they desire to send to this Regt. they can do so and they will be thankfully received.

I have not rode my horse much since I have been here only once in fact but it has been owing mostly to the fact that my secesh saddle was very hard to ride on and rubbed my horses back sore. I have the best horse in the Regt. I was offered $150.00 in gold for him the other day but refused it. I would sell him if I could get enough to suit me. The horse suits me too well to sell him. [I] am glad to hear of the welfare of Maggie and Jessie. [I] cant get a leave of absence to go to Indianapolis. Shall buy me a saddle to-morrow.

You probably see by Ed Allens boys case that Typhoid fever is not so much of a fever as it is an inflammation of a certain portion of the bowels and the peculiar fever a consequence of it & in proportion to the irritation of the bowel so is the fever. But I must close. Write soon.

Yours affectionately
J. D. Benton

P.S. Will you send me a few postage stamps in your next letter? We can't get them here in quantities less than $2.00 worth.

The report is to-day that we are coming home to winter I think it probable.

*   *   *

Camp Douglas
Chicago, Ill.
Nov 4 1862

Dear Father,

I have been expecting a letter from you for several days but thought I would write to-night as I know you want to hear from me as often as possible.

I have just been writing to Maggie a long letter. The hopes of the boys have rather fallen for a day or two as they expected by this time to have been in [New] York State but it seems to have blown over for the present. The rebound of their feelings is like that of an old musket at its discharge all the other way. Still I think that we will be sent to our own state in a short time

same more or less. Things go on in the same style the same thing over every day.

I believe I have not told you how our camp and surroundings are situated. Our camp probably contains a hundred acres of land but there are many troops camped outside including these. I think it would not fall short of two hundred acres of land it is on the prairie and is as level as a house floor with the exceptions of the ditches for its drainage. It is covered with long barracks mostly arranged in squares for the troops, the troops under the charge of the Post Surgeon will not fall far short of 12,000 in number. We are southeast of the city about 4 miles, but the buildings extend all the way down and make it all city. A horse railroad is the communication which run up and down all the time 5 c[en]ts the fare.

Just around the city the land is low prairie and so wet as not to be hardly tillable. Hardly anything is raised for miles around the city, until you get back to higher land which I suppose is beautiful country. Everything is very high here compared with NY State nothing can be bought here unless at double what it is worth. The city is largely inhabited by Germans and old country people and you would think in passing through the streets that every other man got his living by drinking Lager beer and Schnapps.

I am from my position acquainted with nearly if not all the physicians of the different Regts. in camp some of them are men of the best education and some just the other way but in general they are a fine set of men, the best one in camp I think is Frederick Wolf[12], a Bohemian he is a truly scientific man as well as a pleasant companion. He is on the board to examine soldiers for discharge and consequently is at the Post Surgeons office much of the time. He is the surgeon of the Garibaldi Guards, which you remember were fitted out in New York City [and are] perhaps the greatest fighting men in the world. They are dwindled down to 5 or 600, all hard customers.

I have wandered considerable in my letter but I have written as the thoughts occurred. This war in my opinion must close in less than a year. I consider we have our last piles of soldiers in the field and what is done this fall will have a great influence on the issue, if it continues much longer the government is bankrupt and never can recover itself. I know many will differ from me but I am confident of what I say. I guess there is not many subjects

12 Friedrich Wolff was 26 years old when he was mustered in on May 28, 1861, Company F, 39th New York Volunteer Regiment ("the Garibaldi Guards").

that I have not touched upon in this letter but I have written upon the spur of the moment and hope you will excuse all errors. Write as soon as possible & oblige.

Your son
J. D. Benton

*   *   *

Camp Douglas
November 14/62

Dear Father,

I received your letter dated the 10th and it was welcome indeed for I had received no word by letter or other wise from New York over two weeks and I was getting very lonesome in consequence. I have not received a letter from Maggie for a long time but expect to hear from her every day.

Frank, I suppose, is at home by this time and enjoying himself in visiting his friends. I was very anxious to come with him but I cant get a furlough for love or money. If I could have got a furlough I should have had plenty of the first, the latter I dont know about.

I am entirely recovered from my attack of Jaundice. I dont know from experience of my own much about how it feels to be sick but I am satisfied about Jaundice. I was very sick for some time.

The future prospects of this Regt. are very uncertain and whether we will stay here or not is very doubtful we may winter here and may not stay a week, I am of the opinion that we will be moved to some other camp before long. Where I cannot tell. I think that hostilities will cease by spring either by the defeat of the Rebels or by mutual agreement of the parties.

I am now employed in our own Regiment. The Batteries that were under my charge have been assigned physicians so that I had nothing to do so I requested to be sent back to my own Regt. Dr. Vosburgh has arrived and I was very glad to have him come as he is a very fine man. He was in charge of the hospital at Harpers Ferry and did not come along with us at that time.

I was very glad of the stamps you sent me. You inquire about money. The $25.00 you sent was received. I had to pay out $15.00 for a saddle and bridle and had $10.00 left. Uncle Sam makes us board ourselves, still I have eaten a *great many of his rations. Since I was sick I have had my meals in a private family as I thought it was actually necessary to give me health and strength again. Of course not much of the $10.00 is left. We have to pay 10 cts. a piece for washing shirts and everything else in proportion $2.00 per week for board. I am in need of money of course but I have not sent for it for I did not want to burden you so much with my wants and I also expected to receive some pay soon still it has not come and how soon it will I cannot say. If you should send any money or have any sent, do it immediately as we may soon move. Send it as soon as you get this letter or I may not get it.*

Nothing would give me more pleasure than to come home on Christmas with Richardson but it is impossible to tell what may be the circumstances of the case by that time. I shall try to come if possible and make you a visit. I want to see you all as bad perhaps as you do me and would do anything to come home. I suppose Maggie is well and enjoying herself in visiting among her friends and acquaintances. Jessie is without doubt well and growing finely.

Camp Douglas is getting muddy and nasty as the changeable fall weather comes on and probably will be more so before spring. I hope earnestly and trust that we will be relieved from staying here very long and above all that we may draw our pay.

I hear Bradford Cook is married or going to be. (Let the lion lie down with the lamb). Time goes rather slowly but when I hear from home frequently it makes it seem shorter. Write as if we was going to stay, and dont credit any rumors about our coming home until we arrive in Auburn. Write very soon and often telling me all the news.

Yours affectionately,

J. D. Benton
1st asst. surgeon
111 Regt. NY Vols.
Camp Douglas, Chicago, Ill

*   *   *

Camp Douglas
Chicago, Ill
Nov 21, 1862

Dear Father,

Since I last wrote you things have taken a little change, not as concerning the Regt. but myself. I am to be left in charge of about 35 or 40 sick in our hospital, cure them up and send them on to the Regt. and follow at my leisure and I shall try to fetch up at Cato before I get to Washington.

I am rather pleased with staying as the Regt. will go immediately into the field and be at first compelled to endure many hardships, whereas I shall not be obliged to be in any haste in going. I probably shall stay from 2 to 4 or 6 weeks and shall try to get home while Richardson is there. I can either get government transportation or draw mileage of 6 cts. per mile. I think I shall pay my own transportation and take the mileage. I can travel for 2/3 fare and in taking the mileage I can make considerable. The Regt. will probably start on to-morrow or next day. They are busy making preparations and you have no idea the amount of red tape and machinery necessary in taking charge of sick securing their comfort.

It is late and I must close. If you have sent any money it will be safe as I am going to stay. I was afraid it would be lost if I had went with the Regt. I am well, never weighed as much in my life. Write very often.

Your son
J. D. Benton

Do not direct your letters to Camp Douglas, but simply to Chicago and leave off the number of the Regt. as they follow the Regt. if so directed.

*   *   *

On November 19, 1862, the men of the 39th, 111th, 125th, and 126th New York regiments received news they would be exchanged and thereafter serve in the defenses surrounding Washington, D.C., where they would be armed and put into service on the front lines. The news was met with extreme jubilation, for the soldiers believed they would finally get a second chance to redeem themselves after the disgrace of Harpers Ferry.

The regiments arrived in Washington on November 25 and by early December had been assigned to the defenses of the capital near Union Mills and Centreville, Virginia. The regiments were brigaded under Colonel George Frederick D'Utassy and became the Third Brigade, in Silas Casey's division, XXII Corps. They would remain near Centreville, Virginia until June 1863.

*   *   *

Fairfax Seminary, Va.
Dec 7, 1862

Dear Father,

This is the first opportunity that I have had of writing to you since I arrived at this place. We are about eight miles from Washington and in sight of it and two miles from Alexandria which with the Potomac River are in plain view from our camp, which is received the name of Camp Pomeroy. I suppose in honor of our Congressman T. M. Pomeroy.

It would be impossible for me to give you any description that would be accurate but perhaps I can approximate it in a measure. In the first place there is no inhabitants in miles of this place, not a fence to be seen and the timber has all been cut down or nearly so and the hills are left bare of all but the stumps and brush which has been left as it was cut from the trees. Wagon roads run in every conceivable direction across the fields and over the hills and in the distance you can see the chain of fortifications which are the defense of Washington. In front of our camp towards and facing the Potomac is the residence of Bishop Johns, the once Episcopal rebel who had the supervision of the state of Virginia in a moral sense. He fled and left his warm coffee at breakfast the morning Ellsworth was killed in Alexandria. Probably you recollect reading the circumstance at the time. He left a nice house containing everything but his most moveable valuables and it is now regarded and used as United States property. Our Col. has his headquarters in it and the officers mess in his dining room. There is in the house an old piano made in Dresden which was probably considered as an elegant instrument when new. There is also a theological library of probably several hundred volumes although many of the volumes are in appearance somewhat antiquated it would be valuable to a theologian.

The country is a scene of complete desolation and not a spear of grain or anything of the kind is raised in this vicinity for miles around. Our pickets go out 5 or six miles. They go out and stay 48 hours at a time. The Rebels they say have pickets from 15 or 20 miles from here but there is none in this vicinity.

We have just had a severe snow storm. Those knowing the climate say that so severe a one hardly ever occurs. Cold weather only lasts two or three days at a time over there. It comes off warm and pleasant and mud up to your knees. The Regt. is in tents and some of them suffer very much from cold. I was very much disappointed in not being able to come home as I expected. The prospect for pay is more promising then heretofore and if we get paid I shall try to get home and see you all. I am very anxious to come and I guess Maggie would like to see me, as also would all my relatives and friends.

It is getting late and I must close my letter. Write as soon as possible. Direct your letters to 111th Regt. Washington, D.C. and they will reach me. Write soon.

Yours affectionately
James D. Benton

*   *   *

Washington D.C.
Dec 23, 1862

Dear Father,

I have intended to write you for some time past but business and an illness of two or three days have prevented until now.

I am at present at Fairfax Seminary in the hospital, which we occupied while the Regt. was camped here and in which we left several sick which have not yet been moved. The Regt. is located south of here about 3 miles directly down the Potomac and about 2 ½ miles from Alexandria across what is *called Hunting Creek which empties into the Potomac between Alexandria and our camp. It is only about 5 ½ miles down to Mount Vernon[13] from the Regt. and as soon as I can find time I am going to make it a visit. The Regt. is now in [Silas] Caseys Division in a Brigade commanded by Col. Grimshaw acting Brig[adier]. Genl. I think we are in our winter quarters and my opinion will be confirmed if we dont move until the rains come on and make the roads bad. The roads are good now as we have had quite dry weather. The days are pleasant but the nights are very cold.*

The Regt. are occupied in working on Fort Lyon most of the time but occasionally send out pickets. The dome of the Capitol [Building] is in plain view as also Alexandria and the Potomac River. The hills around and west of us covered by forts and camps and intersected & crossed in every conceivable way by wagon roads and paths. This is truly a desolate country not a family as I know of in miles except contrabands who are everywhere in abundance. Years and years will elapse before it can be worth anything to anyone. The times are very hard here in all respects and no prospects of improvement until this war closes.

We have a good building for a hospital for the men not yet removed. It is on a hill with beautiful ground around it with large trees in front but not a sign of cultivation except of the arts of war as back of the house all along the edge of the hill are rifle pits. Many of the trees have been cut down and every day I order one or two cut down for the use of our stoves & fireplaces which latter are very nicely made of marble but the Yankee boot has took the polish off in trying to get his heels higher than his head.

But I have written quite lengthy and must close my wandering letter as it is bedtime. I would like very much to sleep in a good feather bed to-night but I content myself with straw turning over to ease my hip bones occasionally. Content must supply all deficiencies but I am afraid it won't bring Christmas dinner with turkey. But I must stop. Write very often.

Your affectionate Son,
James D Benton

*   *   *

---

13 Located near Alexandria, Virginia, Mount Vernon (constructed in 1757) was the plantation home of George Washington, the first president of the United States.

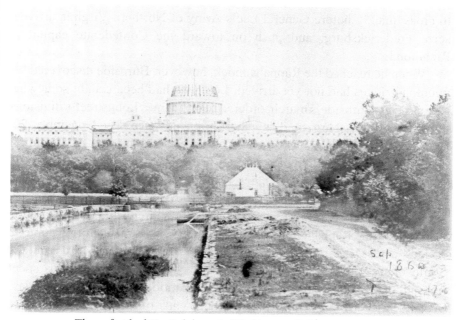

The unfinished Capitol dome in Washington, D.C. *National Archives*

The Army of the Potomac ended 1862 with a devastating loss at the Battle of Fredericksburg. Ambrose Burnside, who had replaced George B. McClellan[14] at the head of the army, answered President Lincoln's call for action by shifting the army quickly to the Rappahannock River. He intended

14 George Brinton McClellan was the former commander of the Army of the Potomac. He graduated second in his West Point Class of 1846, performed well in the War with Mexico in an engineering company, and served overseas as an observer during the Crimean War. President Abraham Lincoln placed McClellan in command of the military forces in and around Washington, where he organized and trained an army of 75,000 men. After his defeat by General Robert E. Lee on the Virginia peninsula outside Richmond during the Seven Days' Battles (June 25 - July 1, 1862), McClellan reorganized the remnants of Major General John Pope's defeated Army of Virginia, forced the South Mountain passes in Maryland, and stopped Lee's invasion at Antietam on September 17, 1862. Though a tactical defeat, the battle was a strategic victory and Lincoln used it as the basis for issuing his Emancipation Proclamation. When McClellan failed to pursue Lee aggressively after Antietam, Lincoln ordered him removed from command on November 5, 1862, and elevated Ambrose Burnside in his place. In 1864, McClellan was the leading Democratic candidate for president but was defeated by Lincoln. In 1877, he received the Democratic nomination for governor of New Jersey, winning the seat by almost 13,000 votes. He died on October 29, 1885 at the age of 58.

to cross quickly before General Lee's Army of Northern Virginia arrived, seize Fredericksburg, and push on toward the Confederate capital at Richmond.

When he reached the Rappahannock, however, Burnside discovered his pontoon bridges had not yet arrived. Lee, who had been caught somewhat off-guard by Burnside's march, ordered two of James Longstreet's divisions toward Fredericksburg to delay the Union advance. By November 22, Longstreet's entire corps was on high ground behind the city. As a result of the delay, the Union would have to cross in the face of the Confederate army. The other Confederate corps under Thomas "Stonewall" Jackson reached Fredericksburg on December 3, marching nearly 175 miles in just 12 days. Robert E. Lee had his entire army and a nearly impregnable position on the hills west of the Rappahannock. On December 11, Burnside threw pontoon bridges across the river under fire while Union batteries fired on the Confederates but failed to fully drive them off. December 12 was spent crossing the river and preparing for the attack to follow. The following day, December 13, Union troops attacked both ends of Lee's lines, but were driven back with heavy losses.[15]

The war had reached a pivotal point. Although Union forces in the Western Theater were experiencing a steady string of successes (the Army of the Cumberland scored a major strategic victory at Stones River in Tennessee during the closing days of 1862 and first day of 1863), the same could not be said for the state of the war in the Eastern Theater.

---

15 The best book available on this topic remains Francis O'Reilly's, *The Fredericksburg Campaign: Winter War on the Rappahannock* (Baton Rouge, LA, 2006).

1863

President Lincoln removed General Burnside from command on January 26, 1863, after cold weather and heavy winter rains brought about the failure of another attempted offensive history has dubbed "The Mud March." The president replaced Burnside with Major General Joseph Hooker, who had worked behind Burnside's back for the elevation to army command.

* * *

Centreville, Va.
January 26, 1863

Dear Father,

It is quite a long time since I wrote you last, nevertheless I could have intended to write many times but it has so happened that I could not. But it is perhaps better late than never.

As you see by the top of my letter we are at Centreville, VA on the sacred soil of the "Old Dominion" and it indeed looks like an old Dominion, nothing about it wears the appearance of youth. You know the location of

Centreville as well as I could tell you suffice it to say that we are about 3 ½ or 4 miles from the stream which is called Bull Run.[1] The nearest point to the stream is in a southwesterly direction, the country between us and it is rolling until within about a mile of it. Then it is rather low and covered by scattering trees and now the wall is very muddy except a corduroy road the Rebels made for artillery that is as good as ever and is made of small trees laid down close together. The main battles took place farther up the creek and it is not considered quite safe to venture there as it is outside our picket lines, but I shall try it some day. At the point I went which is called Mitchels Ford, are Rebel intrenchments thrown up on the opposite side all along the creek and the remains of masked Batteries. I also [see] the Manassas Rail Road Bridge, and the place where Gen. [John] Pope[2] burnt his stores. A person frequently sees clothes, old gun shells scattered over the ground. This was all to be seen at Mitchels Ford.

No doubt you have an idea of Centreville but I am confident it is not correct, there is not over 8 or 10 houses at most standing and a few in ruins. They are as all Virginia houses, whitewashed and they are in very old style [with] huge chimneys built on the outside of each and the very personification of loneliness in the present and of "Niggers" and whiskey in the past. The whole land is covered by ruins of camps and fortifications. I have not seen a fence since I left Alexandria, the nearest to it was a row of posts where there used to be one before the war.

1   The area, about 28 miles outside Washington D.C., was the site of the July 21, 1861 Battle of Bull Run (or Manassas), the first major engagement of the Civil War. The Union army of about 32,000 men was under Brigadier General Irvin McDowell, who attacked a similar sized Confederate force led by Pierre G. T. Beauregard, who was reinforced during the battle by the arrival of men from the Shenandoah Valley under General Joseph E. Johnston. The battle ended when the Union army was routed from the field. The Second Battle of Bull Run (or Manassas) was fought on some of the same ground on August 28-30, 1862, between Union Major General John Pope's Army of Virginia and Confederate General Robert E. Lee's Army of Northern Virginia. The battle routed Pope from the field and paved the way for the first Confederate invasion of the North.

2   John Pope was born March 16, 1822 in Louisville, Kentucky, graduated West Point in 1842 and won brevets for gallantry in the Mexican War. Appointed a Brigadier General of Volunteers on June 4, 1861. Promoted to Major General on March 22, 1862. In June of that same year he was given command of all forces in the East (Army of Virginia) except those under Major General George B. McClellan on the Peninsula. His men were designated to protect Washington D.C. He failed at the 2nd Battle of Bull Run and was put in the Department of the Northwest where he served during the Sioux uprising in Minnesota. He retired from the army in 1886. Died September 23, 1892.

Our Regt. lie[s] on a hill just behind and not over 100 rods from Centreville. We are between two fortifications built by the Rebels and in which the "Quaker Guns"[3] thundered forth their dignified silence at [George B.] McClellans army their places are filled with more noisy successors. No artillery near us except light [artillery] until we reach Fairfax Court House and it is heavier as we go toward the defenses of Washington in which the size is enormous. We are under the same Dutassy as at Harpers Ferry but a genuine Brig. Genl has now taken command, his name is Brig. Genl [Alexander] Hays[4], Dutassy is only acting Brig. We are brigaded with the same Regts that we were with at Harpers Ferry[5].

The sight is splendid from our camp. We can see far into Rebeldom, the Blue Ridge [Mountains] and Thoroughfare Gap are in plain sight and we could see this morning the snow upon the mountains far off to the west. The valley through which Bull Run and Cub Run passes are down below us apparently but a short distance but in fact a long one.

But I must close my letter at least the topographical part of it. I am in the best of health and weigh 15 pounds more than ever in my life. The health of the Regt. is gradually improving and we hope will continue to do so. Frank is well, I received a letter from Maggie yesterday and one from Heman to-day, [I] am glad to hear of their welfare. Write to me often, I most forgot we are going to be paid in a few days. Give me the news and remember me to all my friends. My love to Ma and the family generally.

Your affectionate son
J. B. Benton

3   A Quaker gun is a wooden log painted black to deceive the enemy. The name derived from the Religious Society of Friends ("Quakers") who were opposed to war and violence.

4   Born July 8, 1819 in Franklin, Pennsylvania, Hays entered West Point in 1840 and graduated in the bottom third of his class four years later. He won a brevet for gallantry in the Mexican War but resigned in 1848 to engage in the iron business and then to California to prospect for gold. At the outbreak of the Civil War, Hays reentered the army as colonel of the 63rd Pennsylvania (and as captain in the Regular Army with the 16th Infantry). He served well in early 1862 on the Virginia peninsula, was severely wounded at Second Bull Run that August, promoted to brigadier general on September 29, and posted to the defenses of Washington D.C. until June 1863. After recovering from his wound, he was assigned to command the 2nd Brigade in the 3rd Division, II Corps, which he led at Gettysburg July 1-3, 1863. Hays was killed in the Wilderness on May 5, 1864.

5   The brigade consisted of the 39th, 111th, 125th, and 126th New York volunteer regiments under Colonel George L. Willard.

*   *   *

Joe Hooker demonstrated an amazing ability for organization and leadership. With help from several key subordinates including Chief of Staff Dan Butterfield, Hooker rebuilt the army from the ground up. He instituted critical logistical, ordnance, and administrative reforms and insisted his troops receive good care and undergo tough inspections and battle drills. Hooker issued promotions and furloughs on a merit basis, launched a series of raids large and small, streamlined the army's command and control, created a new cavalry corps, and ushered in a better military intelligence organization. Morale skyrocketed. Some of his soldiers took to calling the winter interlude "The Army of the Potomac's Valley Forge."[6]

*   *   *

Centreville, Va.
Feb. 18, 1863

Dear Father,

It has been a very long time since I have heard from you and I am at somewhat of a loss to account for so long a silence. I have written several letters to you since I received your last. Things remain about the same as usual and there is nothing remarkable or new in our camp except perhaps a flurry of snow last night which the boys improve by snowballing. The duties of the camp is mostly doing picket duty which is not as hard as it was because the Garibaldi Guards (39th N.Y.)[7] and the 125th N.Y.[8] do their equal share so

---

6 For a complete look at Hooker's transformation of the army, see Albert Z. Conner and Chris Mackowsi, *Seizing Destiny: The Army of the Potomac's "Valley Forge" and the Civil War Winter that Saved the Union* (Savas Beatie, 2016).

7 The Garibaldi Guards (39th New York) was organized and recruited in New York City by Colonel George D'Utassy and mustered into service for three years at Washington D.C. on June 6, 1861. This unique command consisted of three companies of Germans, three of Hungarians, one of Swiss, one of Italians, one of Frenchmen, one of Spaniards, and one of Portuguese. During its service the regiment lost 9 officers and 269 enlisted men.

8 Colonel John A. Griswold was authorized on July 28, 1862 to raise the regiment (125th NY) in Rensselaer County. Upon his resignation, Colonel George L. Willard succeeded him

it only comes to our Regt. once in two days. They go out and stay 48 hours each. The pickets extend from Blackburns Ford to or nearly to the Stone Bridge. I believe it takes 150 men. They are mostly stationed on the north bank of Bull Run.

We have now about an inch and a half of snow but it probably will go tomorrow it never stays long here. The sickness in the Regt. is declining having only 26 [men] in hospital. We have received our pay for two months and in 4 or 5 weeks will probably receive pay again. I took Major Austin the Paymaster to Washington in an ambulance and he said he was assured by the Department that we should receive our money regularly hereafter.

There is no movement of the armies on either side in this immediate vicinity and probably there is no force of Rebels of any size near us at present. Occasionally guerilla parties approach our lines and skirmish with our cavalry pickets but they are quite cautious. Col. Windham perhaps you saw by the papers went out with quite a force from Fairfax C[ourt] H[ouse] and went all around through rebeldom, his force passed through this place. I saw them go out. It did not avail much I believe. Such raids do not affect the general result to any amount.

You can but form a poor estimate of the injury the war has done in this country poor enough at the best although under proper cultivation might be made very fruitful. The boys from our vicinity are mostly well. Alson Chase has been sick with fever but I cured him (homeopathically) large fever, large doses of Aconite. But it is very late and I must done, we have to get up very early, long before daylight. I trust I may hear from you soon. Is ma and yourself well[?] Give my love to all. Goodbye

Affectionately,

J. D. Benton

*   *   *

---

on August 15, 1862. The regiment was organized at Troy, New York and mustered into service for three years on August 27-29, 1862. It was mustered out June 5, 1865, near Alexandria, Virginia. The regiment lost 16 officers and 227 enlisted men.

Centreville, Va.
Feb. 28, 1863
Dear Father and Mother,

You can hardly imagine how very welcome your letter was to me. I had just written a letter or partly written it to Pa in which I set forth my disappointment and anxiety in not hearing from you. I had also written to Maggie concerning it when lo it comes and I have read it three or four times already.

No one without experience in the army can conceive how delightful it is for the soldier to hear from his friends and relatives. The rush for letters among the soldiers is only perhaps equaled by a bayonet charge on a Battery. The barrel of articles sent to Co[mpany] H by the Cato ladies reached us last night in safety and in good order. I shall notice it in the Auburn paper but wish not to claim it as my own composition as it is to be written for others. I shall write to Laura to-morrow for as it is her first absence from home without doubt she is very lonesome and would like to hear from me.

The last day of every two months we are inspected and mustered for pay and to-day was the regular day so as you might say we have been under arms all day or nearly all. The Paymaster said that we would receive our pay regularly hereafter i.e.: every two months. So we will be paid again in three or four weeks and I shall be able then to send home about $400.00. I have many times indeed been in want of money but have got along very well. I have been for a month or so without a red [?] still I felt as well as if I was spending a dollar a day.

We are at Centreville about 22 miles from Washington as near as I can estimate for what inhabitants there [say]. [They cant tell themselves at least they all give various distances when asked. The direction is almost due west a trifle southerly and about direct west from Alexandria. Four miles south of us or nearly so is the present terminus of the Orange and Alexandria Railroad. The cars would run farther but the Rebels dont like to have them. Transportation by this road to Washington is generally obtained but being strictly [a] military road a transportation pass has to be obtained from the Brig. Genl. Hays. But the trip on horseback is made most generally by those who have horses.

Where I went I rode in an ambulance and took back the Paymaster and his trunk of greenbacks [dollars]. About our quarters (we dont call them winter quarters) they are simply cotton tents about eight feet square for privates and officers have larger. Mine is about ten by twelve I think very convenient as to size. Three of us inhabit it. I prefer a medium sized one as it is more favorable as to warmth than a large one. I have a tick filled with straw but I dare not throw [away] the straw, which is rather ancient for fear I might not be able to get any more. It is very comfortable however.

[I] am sorry to confess to being lousey, but I have captured ten or a dozen on several different occasions but I find that they range over the high in authority as well as the low.[9] I have washed myself all over and found them the same day at night so friendly are they. Each tent has a stove and I have not been uncomfortable except perhaps one night.

As I have consumed so much paper I can hardly be able to say much about the city of "magnificent distances" nor have I seen many of the great men, except Sumner and Hale. I saw one day the Senate in session but was unable to stay to find out who were and who were not the celebrities. I was intending to call on President Lincoln but before the time of day in which he received visitors. I was compelled to leave. Still I have been at the White House. Anyone and everyone is received and welcomed there on certain days and at certain hours of the day or anytime if he is not engaged with public affairs.

For a day or two when we first came I stayed with some sick men in the city being delayed in getting transportation across the river and I visited several places of interest viz the Capitol, the patent office, the post office and above all the Smithsonian Institute which latter was of more interest except perhaps the Capitol than all else. The two being a different quality of mental enjoyment. The Capitol is an architectural wonder indeed but the Institute is a compilation of natures most beautiful specimens from every part of the known world and from every kingdom of creation. Two days time cannot fully examine a 100th part of its curiosities arranged in perfect order as they are. I need not try to give you any idea of its magnitude for it is beyond the power of communication on paper.

I may reiterate in my letters something that I have said before as I cannot always tell what I wrote you last. Ma says she likes long letters and I think I have done very well this time. I desire very much to come home before or during this coming summer and I will if the powers that be will let me. I have

9 Lice was a common problem for soldiers in the field.

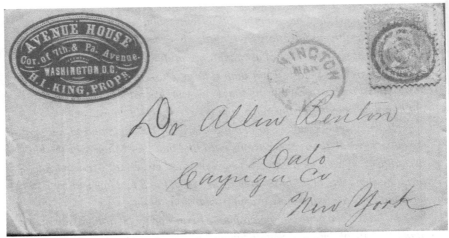

Envelope from one of James's letters home to his father. *Benton Family*

not space to describe our winter but suffice it to say that it has been very mild. I will describe it more fully in my next.

I wish Ma would write in every letter. Write soon.

Your affectionate son,
J. D. Benton

P.S. Direct to Washington as usual, put on the NY Vols and number of Regt. always JDB

*   *   *

Sunday March 1st, 1863
[Centreville, Va.]

Went to bed as usual. Before I went to sleep [I] heard that a telegraph dispatch from Brig. Gen. Hays was received that we must be on the alert as the enemy had been seen near and around the Blackburns Ford. At 12 o'clock precisely the long row was beat and the whole force in Centreville was out in a short time and formed in line of battle. After standing out in the rain about 2 hours the Regts. returned to await more demonstrations. It was splendid to hear on the night air the alarm run along several miles of picket lines at 10 o'clock to day nothing has occurred. We are prepared to give them a warm reception.

The 111th I dont think will ever surrender again and that idea is generally prevalent in it. They would have fought like demons last night, of course the medical corps; Dr. Vosburgh and I were armed with the necessary articles and were on hand punctually. It starts a little chill occasionally to hear the long roll at dead of night and get out bandages and instruments to bind up the wounds. It makes a fellow feel rather curious at first but he soon is accustomed to it. It would scare a novice out of his senses to hear the officers call out their men the long roll continuing to beat until the line is formed and the hurry and tumult in the midnight darkness. Whether we are to be disturbed or not remains to be seen.

Good Bye

Your son
J.D. Benton

*   *   *

Centreville, Va.
April 5, 1863

Dear Father and Mother,

I received your very welcome letter last night and proceed directly to reply.

War and politics receive but a small share of our attention and I have often thought how remarkable it was that political matters were as little thought of as they are in the army. You hear nothing of it unless the condemnation of the infamous copperheadism[10] of the north. This detestable course of a few northern politicians create the utmost indignation in the army that while they are enduring the hardships of rain and snow, depriving

---

10 Republicans called Northern Peace Democrats "Copperheads," because they were opposed to a vigorous prosecution of the war and favored negotiation and compromise to end the war, restore the Union, and keep slavery intact.

themselves of the comforts that they now so greatly appreciate, insidious and wily traitors lie back in the rear ready to frustrate if possible them to greater exertions and in my opinion the opening of good weather will witness the most terrible carnage this continent ever saw.

I am glad you have a license to practice and I would have my pay for all I did it is not right in respect to other physicians to do business for nothing. I forgot to send you the vaccine matter and will enclose some in this letter. I sent home by Ira Dudley my forceps and my amputating case. If we move I cant possibly take care of anything, only what I can carry on my horse and my clothes will be all I want. We have plenty of instruments and I have not the slightest need of them.

I was awakened the other night about twelve o'clock by an order from General Hays by an order to go out to the picket lines. I went immediately it was on or near what is called the Warrenton turnpike about two miles from camp, it appears that a picket in making his patrol from one post to another lost his way it being covered with low pine brush and got outside the line and as he came towards the post he was halted and probably being a little frightened, he partially concealed himself behind a bush, the sentinel fired supposing it to be a rebel. If he had approached openly he would have been safe. What I speak of more particularly is the character of the wound he was struck in the left breast some distance above the nipple the [minié] ball[11] hitting the rib and being partly checked by his clothes and suspender it glanced outward keeping in the flesh passed over the bone in the arm and came out on the backside, its course almost a semicircle if it had went straight he would have been killed of course. I brought him in an ambulance and dressed his wound he is doing well. Dr. Vosburgh is now a thorough convert to the virtues of Aconite and the use of any other Febrifuge of that class is now out of use in our hospital entirely. No case has died in which we used it.

I guess I have run my paper empty and will close. I have no fault to find only the time between your letters. Write often.

---

11 The minié ball is named after its 1849 French inventor, Captain Claude-Etienne Minié. The soft one-ounce lead conical bullet was grooved so that when fired, the round expanded into the rifling of the barrel and exited the barrel spinning at a much higher velocity than a regular musket ball. This also made it much more accurate. Minie balls often shattered bone and thus required amputation.

My love to all

Your son
J.D. Benton

I wish if Elder Garfield wants to rent my place that you would rent it to him for what you think it is worth and if he pays anything down take it and use it I would have some advance pay.

*   *   *

In April of 1863 Joseph Hooker set out to defeat his Confederate opponent in north Central Virginia. His plan was a good one. Hooker first launched a massive cavalry strike behind the Confederate army, maintained a large diversionary force opposite Fredericksburg to fool the Southerners he was still in position, and then marched westward to slip around his enemy's left flank in a move that surprised everyone including General Lee himself.[12]

The early stages of the Chancellorsville Campaign could not have unfolded more to his liking. Lee, however, figured out Hooker's plan and divided his army, keeping a small part opposite Fredericksburg and rushing the balance westward to meet the Union advance. The move stunned Hooker, who had anticipated that Lee would retreat from his Rappahannock line.

Falling back into the tangle of the Wilderness, Hooker remained in place while Lee divided his force once more, sending General Jackson's corps

12 Robert Edward Lee was born January 19, 1807 to Henry and Ann Carter Lee. He graduated second in his West Point Class of 1825 without a single demerit to his name. During his long and stellar service as a staff officer during the Mexican War, Lee learned many of the skills he would put to use during the Civil War. Lee joined the Confederate cause after Virginia seceded from the Union on April 19, 1861. After turning in a mixed performance in western Virginia and along the south Atlantic coast, Lee was brought to Richmond by President Jefferson Davis as a military advisor. When Joe Johnston fell gravely wounded on May 31, 1862 just outside Richmond, Lee was installed as the Eastern army's commander the next day. At the head of the Army of Northern Virginia, Lee turned and defeated General McClellan in the Seven Days' Battles, marched north and defeated General Pope at Second Manassas, fought to a tactical draw in Maryland at Sharpsburg (Antietam), and inflicted severe defeats against the enemy at Fredericksburg and Chancellorsville. Despite his decisive defeat at Gettysburg, Lee would remain in command until the end of the war. After the war, Lee became president of Washington College (soon to be Washington and Lee University), and died on October 12, 1870.

around Hooker's right in what is now considered one of the war's greatest surprise attacks. Although the Army of the Potomac survived the blow and was in a strong defensive position, Hooker eventually conceded defeat and withdrew his army despite outnumbering the Confederates two to one. Hooker had lost his nerve, but Lee would lose Stonewall Jackson a week later when he died after suffering a mortal wound inflicted by friendly fire.[13]

*   *   *

Centreville, Va.
May 31, 1863

Dear Father,

I wrote you a letter yesterday and was about to send it but before I could send it I was gratified by the appearance of Maggie; they had a very pleasant journey indeed and got through safely.

I am now detached from the Regt. and am placed in charge of the Brigade hospital the whole concern is in my hands as far as the hospital is concerned. The office of Brigade Surgeon is abolished and all rank as surgeons or assistants. The Chief Med[ical] officer of the Brigade or as I might better say the Senior acts as Brigade Surgeon and he has put me in charge of the Brigade hospital of course subject to his orders.

We have a good house for this country and I and Maggie have all the room that we wish. I have had a bedroom fixed up with home made furniture but Maggie thinks it very comfortable indeed and she is well pleased with her accommodations. I shall have her stay a long time if the Brigade makes no distant move. All she is troubled about is Jessie but we both know that she will have the best of care and that makes us perfectly contented. I shall keep her as long as she can be persuaded to stay.

We have very good board in the hospital but not quite as good as in camp. However, here it costs me nothing to live and there $3.00 per week and I can forego many luxuries for that. The sick men are much pleased with having Maggie here and she sits and talks with them and it does them a great deal of good. One fellow said, "it was such a treat to have a woman come and

---

13 See Stephen W. Sears, *Chancellorsville* (Houghton Mifflin, 1996), for a good general history of the Chancellorsville campaign.

sit and talk with him." They are very grateful for every attention and in no respect shall they be neglected if I can prevent it. Maggie was going to write to-day but she thought that this would do for us both. We have just returned from a horseback ride out to the picket line my horse is very gentle and Maggie can go all she wishes.

The rumor to-night is that a raid has been made on Catletts Station down on the [Orange and Alexandria] R[ail] R[oad] toward Warrenton but the truth is not exactly reliable as yet.

I shall have to close my letter now. I thought you would be anxious to hear of Maggies safety. We unite in sending our love to all. Good Bye

As Ever Yours
J.D. Benton

Direct as heretofore

*   *   *

Centreville, Va
June 13, 1863

Dear Parents,

We received your letter to-day and was very glad indeed for we had not heard from home since Maggie came and we were of course anxious to know how you all got along. Maggie intended to write but as I was going to she concluded that mine would answer for both. She is naturally anxious about Jessie and thinks that she must come home soon but I want her to stay as long as we are in our present position. If we were to move of course she would be obliged to go home but as long as we remain here there is to me a great pleasure in having her with me.

I think she enjoys herself very much. We have frequent rides on horseback. The other evening about 3 o'clock PM we started and went down to Blackburns Ford on Bull Run and from there around the picket lines to the Warrenton road and thence home making a ride of nearly ten miles and it was to her a very interesting one. She is a capital rider and like all women "hard on a horse" and sets firm in her saddle. She has had one baulk with her and another fall down but she hung on so I think she is safe.

Things go on in the same old style and nothing new has taken place in fact "all is quiet on the Potomac." Tell Jessie that her Ma has a nice rattlebox for her and is going to bring a nice present when she comes. Tell her to be a good girl and mind Gramma. We see by the papers that Vicksburg[14] [Mississippi] is still in "status quo" and we feel much anxiety concerning it. It is also reported that Gen. [Robert E.] Lee has made a movement and there is some anticipation of a raid in to "My Maryland" and Pennsylvania.

We hope it is not so and if it is he will have Gen. [Joseph] Hooker[15] at his rear and he will march more than six miles a day I know. We unite in sending our love to all and wish you to write oftener of late. Remember us to all our friends and believe us ever.

Your Affectionate Children
JD & Maggie Benton

*   *   *

Recognizing the need for another change, a frustrated Lincoln relieved Hooker and elevated V Corps commander Major General George Gordon Meade to take his place at the head of the Army of the Potomac. When he did

---

14 Vicksburg, Mississippi, was an important port on the Mississippi River, 130 miles of which remained in Southern hands between Vicksburg and Port Hudson, Louisiana. Capturing both places was essential to Union strategy, for it would allow the uninterrupted passage of troops and supplies downriver and isolate Confederate states west of it. Vicksburg was heavily reinforced with artillery along the riverfront, and extensive trench works and forts on the land side. In October of 1862, Maj. Gen. Ulysses S. Grant began military operations against Vicksburg. By June 1863 he was besieging the river port, and after a long siege it surrendered on July 4. The Confederate defeat at Gettysburg on July 3, followed by the fall of Vicksburg the next day was a double blow from which the South could not recover.

15 Massachusetts native Joseph Hooker (November 13, 1814-October 31, 1879) graduated in the middle of his West Point Class of 1837, served as a staff officer in the Mexican War, and won several brevets up to lieutenant colonel for gallant conduct. He was commissioned brigadier general of volunteers in August 1861, and went on to fight well at the Seven Days' Battles, Second Bull Run, Antietam, and Fredericksburg. After he was relieved in late June, he was ordered to the Western Theater, where he led a corps at Chattanooga and captured Lookout Mountain and fought well during the Atlanta campaign. When he was passed over for command of the Army of the Tennessee, he asked to be relieved of command. He exercised departmental command until his retirement in 1868 as a major general.

so on June 28, the army was moving north in search of the elusive Lee, who had assumed the strategic offensive and was already operating deep in Pennsylvania.[16]

On June 25, 1863 the 111th New York and the rest of the brigade joined with the Army of the Potomac and was designated the Third Brigade of the Third Division, Second Corps. The opposing armies met at Gettysburg, in southeastern Pennsylvania on the first day of July. For three days (July 1-3) the armies fought the largest battle of the war. By the time the fighting ended, nearly 51,000 men had been killed, wounded, captured, or were missing from both armies.

The 111th New York, under the command of Colonel Clinton D. MacDougall, part of George Willard's brigade, arrived at Gettysburg early in the morning on July 2. The regiment took up a position along the right center of the Union battle line near Ziegler's Grove on Cemetery Ridge. Late that afternoon, the Confederates launched a major attack against the left flank of the Union line, which was held by Dan Sickles' III Corps. The heavy assaults began collapsing Sickles' front around the Peach Orchard salient and rolled northward until they struck all along Cemetery Ridge.

Thousands of Union troops were rushed south to reinforce the III Corps including the 111th, which numbered about 390 men (two of its companies were not on the field). The regiment helped other Union commands repulse Confederate Brig. Gen. William Barksdale's Mississippi brigade, though Willard was killed during the counterattack. The fighting on July 2 afforded the New Yorkers the chance to prove their bravery, courage, and fighting

16 George Gordon Meade (born on December 31, 1815, in Cadiz, Spain) graduated 19th out of 56 in his West Point Class of 1831. He resigned from the army for several years but returned in 1842, and served well in the Mexican War as an engineer. On August 31, 1861, he was promoted to brigadier general and given command of a brigade of the Pennsylvania Reserves. Meade fought well with McClellan on the Virginia Peninsula during the Seven Days' Battles, and Second Bull Run. Promoted to division command, he fought with Hooker's I Corps at South Mountain, Antietam, and Fredericksburg. Elevated to lead the V Corps, Meade saw but little action at Chancellorsville and was with his corps marching north when given command of the Army of the Potomac, which he led to victory at Gettysburg. From May 1864 until the end of the war he fought under the shadow of U. S. Grant, who moved with the army in the field. At the close of the Civil War in 1865, Meade was assigned to various departments and the Military Division of the Atlantic. He died November 6, 1872 in Philadelphia from pneumonia. Meade still awaits a good biography. Until then, see Tom Huntington, *Searching for George Gordon Meade: The Forgotten Victor of Gettysburg* (Stackpole, 2013).

ability, all of which had been doubted since their surrender at Harpers Ferry during the fall of 1862.[17]

General Lee decided to attack the Union right-center the following day, July 3, in what is popularly known as Pickett's Charge. A massive artillery barrage opened before the the the infantry attack, its purpose to soften the enemy positions and silence Northern artillery. During the cannonade—the largest in America up to that time—the 111th New York was posted about 100 yards behind the Abram Brian house not far from their original position the previous day. In the middle of the bombardment, the New Yorkers moved forward to help bolster the Union line. Numbering around 180 men, they occupied a vacant part of the line just north of the 12th New Jersey.

A short time later, perhaps 12,000 Confederate infantry advanced across the open fields toward Cemetery Ridge. The 111th engaged the enemy once they drew within small arms range, and some members moved out from behind the stone wall to fire into the exposed left flank of the enemy. The failed attack signified the end of the long bloody battle.

Of the more than 200 infantry Union regiments that fought at Gettysburg, only two regiments suffered a higher number of men killed than the 111th New York. Its total losses included 58 killed, 177 wounded, and 14 missing, for a total of 249 men.

The staggering number of wounded and injured created an immediate need for places to care for these unfortunate men. Nearly every available barn, shed, stable, schoolhouse, and private residence was put to use. During and after the battle, division and corps hospitals sprang up behind the long Union line, while regimental medical staffs established field depots or dressing stations during the battle as close to their respective commands as possible.[18]

As an assistant surgeon with the 111th New York, Dr. Benton was likely stationed at the Catherine Guinn farm just 150 yards behind the Union line

---

17 For an outstanding tactical history of the fighting along Cemetery Ridge, including the role of the 111th New York, see David L. Shultz and Scott L. Mingus Sr., *The Second Day at Gettysburg: The Attack and Defense of Cemetery Ridge, July 2, 1863* (Savas Beatie, 2015).

18 The best book about the handling of the wounded and dead remains Greg Coco's *A Strange and Blighted Land. Gettysburg—The Aftermath of a Battle* (Thomas Publications, 1995; reprint, Savas Beatie, 2017).

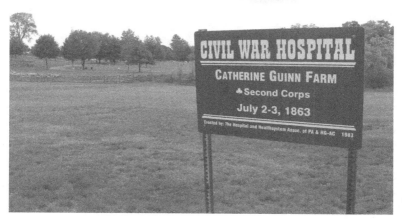

The site of the field hospital where James Benton labored. *Author*

on Cemetery Ridge along the east side of the Taneytown Road.[19] Unfortunately, Dr. Benton was overwhelmed with work treating the wounded and had little time to write during this period.

*   *   *

Hospital 3d Division 2d Corps
July 27, 1863

Dear Parents,

I have wished many times to write to you but my time and facilities for writing have been very limited since the battle [of Gettysburg]. I also knew that you would hear of my safety and welfare by the letters I wrote to Maggie

---

19 The Catherine Guinn farm was just south of the present-day National Cemetery. Unfortunately the farm and buildings were torn down after the war, and much of the land today is a parking lot.

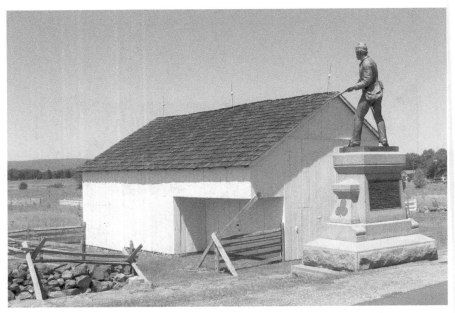

111th New York monument at Gettysburg, looking northwest (above)
and looking east (on facing page). *Author*

and by her letters here all the particulars that I could tell in a letter direct to you.

It is impossible for me to give any adequate description by writing of the terrible engagement through which we have passed and I rather reserve the tale of horrors until I can describe it in person. Of course the surgeons were all busy and have been until now. When the "Army of the Potomac" moved in pursuit of Lee, I was detailed to remain as an assistant to Dr. McAbee with one other of our Division forming an operating board. Dr. McAbee[20] is the Chief Surgeon of our Division and for over a week I had the opportunity of assisting in hundreds of very important operations and in consequence my mind is impressed with many items relating to surgery that I should not have gained had I gone on with the Regt.

I should judge that we have now about 600 wounded in our corps including many Rebels perhaps 200 in number who receive the same attention as our own men. This is only one corps and considering the fact that

20 Dr. McAbee was with the 4th Ohio, which was part of the 3rd Division, II Corps.

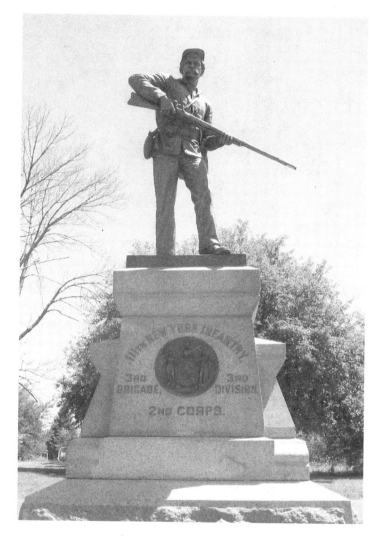

there are seven corps and that every day or two a train containing from 4 to 500 wounded sent away to different hospitals you can form but a slight conception of the number injured in the engagement. The fact is no idea of the Army of the Potomac can be formed until one has seen it. Maggie can give you a little idea of it but she saw only about half of it while at Centreville.

I have not heard from home since I left Centreville just about one month ago and do not know even now whether Maggie arrived home in safety but presume she did still I am anxious to hear. I wrote her my whereabouts as I went along wherever I could do so.

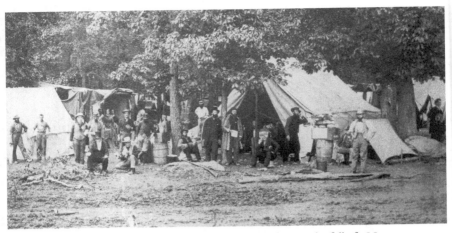

A 2nd Corps hospital near Rock Creek, Gettysburg in the fall of 1863. *NPS*

We have been very uncertain how long we were to stay at Gettysburg but I am inclined to think we may stay a week or two longer and I want you all to write immediately so that I may hear how you all are and the news of interest. I see that I have almost filled my sheet and must soon stop. I want some money sent to me while here as I have only 15 cents in my exchequer and need more immediately. I want $15.00 or $20.00.

I shall probably join the Regt. by the overland route on horseback and must have some funds for grub &c. If it is sent immediately I shall receive it. It takes about three days for a letter to reach here.

I must close. Give my love to my friends in Cato and Ira. Write me as soon as possible and tell me the news. Kiss my little girl and believe me.

Ever your Affectionate Son

James D. Benton
1st asst surgeon
111th Regt
Hospital 3d Division 2d Corps
Near Gettysburg Pa

* * *

July 28, 1863

I have just received an order to leave for the Regt. in the morning and if the money has not been sent dont send it. If it is on the way I will leave arrangements so as to get it sent on to me.

Good Bye
JDB

*   *   *

Arlington Heights, Va.
Washington D.C.
August 4, 1863

Dear Father,

It has been a very long time since you have heard from me with the exception of one letter which I believe I wrote you from Gettysburg Pa. As you see by this I am at Washington.

For two months past two companies of our Regt. have been on detached duty along Orange and Alexandria R.R. and when I arrived here I found them guarding a camp of contrabands at Arlington Heights and I not being very well stopped with them. We are within 20 rods[21] of the famous Arlington House, the dwelling of the Rebel Gen. Lee, the house where he did not eat his Fourth of July dinner as he predicted a month or so since. His dinner on that day was no doubt eaten in a far different place and under very peculiar circumstances viz on the "skedaddle" from Penn[sylvania], with a fire in his rear.[22]

---

21 One rod is about 16.6 feet.

22 Lee's Gettysburg retreat was punctuated with fighting all the way to the Potomac River, which was not readily fordable. He had no choice but to throw up powerful entrenchments and wait for the water to go down so he could cross, which he did on the night of July 13-14, 1863. For the best treatment of this part of the campaign, see Eric J. Wittenberg, J. David Petruzzi, and Michael Nugent, *One Continuous Fight: The Retreat from Gettysburg and the Pursuit of Lee's Army of Northern Virginia, July 4 - 14, 1863* (Savas Beatie, 2011).

Our Regiment is at Warrenton Junction and is said to have been lately detached from the 2nd Army Corps. We all hope it is so. I received my pay to-day for the two past months viz May & June. They owe me for July and this month as far as it is past. I sent to the care of Geo[rge] Rich to Weedsport [NY] $175.00 and in writing to Maggie to-day, I forgot to send the receipt as it might be necessary to get the money so I enclose it in this and you will please hand it to him and he will get the money.

But I must stop for the present I have had no letter from home for over a month. Write soon. Give my love to all. Good Bye

Your Affectionate Son
J. D. Benton

*   *   *

Camp near Elkton Va.
Aug. 16th 1863

Dear Father,

I have for a long time past been so circumstanced that I could not write to you near as frequently as I many times wished I could and when I did write my conveniences were such that I could not make my communications very agreeable or interesting to you.

You doubtless have heard many descriptions of the terrible strife at Gettysburg and for that reason I shall remain silent on that subject. Suffice it to say that no imagination can torture itself into anything like the reality.

I left the hospital at Gettysburg on the 29th of July under orders to report to my Regt. with the least possible delay. I had previously picked up a wounded horse & a saddle, which I used on the journey, & it was a long journey indeed to ride. I was accompanied by our estimable Chaplain whose company relieved the irksomeness of the long ride very much. For a week before I started I was sick with bloody dysentery and during the ride I was troubled with it and I had to stop by the roadside frequently to heave up my internals. I persevered until I arrived at Washington [where] I rested over one night with Capt Irvin Squires of the 9th [New York] Artillery and got rested considerably.[23]

At Washington I procured a leave to lay off of duty for ten days. I stayed eight and then started for the Regt. I found them located six or eight miles southeast of Warrenton Junction. The morning I arrived they were moving camp and I met them on the march. Our Regt. is now a pitiful sight. It was almost annihilated but what is left of it are proud of their deeds and whenever they go into a fight again blood will be spilled.

At the time of this writing and since last night we were under orders to be ready to march at a moments notice and our brigade commander tells me that he thinks we will move before night. The question most naturally arises where are we going? I can only give what I hear and my own opinion based upon it. There are troops going to Alexandria by the thousands constantly on the Rail Road of course there is no use for them there consequently that cannot be their final destination. My opinions, and I think there are good reasons for them, is that we will bring up at one of 3 places - 1st Charleston - 2nd North Carolina - 3rd the Peninsula, of which one of the two latter in view of all the circumstances appears most plausible to me. If the forces under Beauregard[24] at Charleston are defeated they doubtless would endeavor to effect a junction with Lee and overwhelm the Army of the Potomac unless they were placed in [a] more favorable position than now.

The fact that Genl. Meade has just joined the army from a visit at Washington and the movement of troops in so great numbers makes me think that a different course will now be pursued at least from a different point. It is the prevalent opinion here that we are going south somewhere. If we could

---

23 Squires was 32 when he mustered in as captain of Company K, 138th New York Infantry on September 8, 1862. He was wounded on June 1 and 7, 1864 at Cold Harbor, Virginia and was a major when he was discharged for disability on May 15, 1865. Colonel Joseph Welling recruited the 138th New York in Auburn, New York and mustered it into service for three years on September 8-9, 1862. The men were rushed to Washington and served there as both infantry and artillerymen. That December it was redesignated 9th New York Heavy Artillery, and some of the companies reinforced the Army of the Potomac in 1864 and saw significant action around Petersburg and with the Army of the Shenandoah in the Valley. It was mustered out July 6, 1865 at Washington D.C. https://dmna.ny.gov/ historic/reghist/civil/artillery/9thHeavyArty/9thHeavyArtyMain.htm, last accessed on September 18, 2017.

24 Pierre Gustave Toutant Beauregard was a Confederate general in command at Charleston. He led the Southern army to a victory at First Manassas (Bull Run) in July 1861, fought in the Western Theater, and was finally sent to Charleston, where he served well.

surround Richmond from the south and cut off their supplies, they could not last long for they could get nothing from the country north of the Rappahannock [River]. I am impressed that this idea has been resolved upon by the Cabinet in consultation with Genl. Meade.[25]

I have nearly filled my paper and must soon stop. The draft I suppose grinds rather hard with many of the inhabitants of Cayuga [County, NY] but it is no more severe for a drafted man than a volunteer both have to obey orders. The weather is excessively warm, hot I should say but the nights are getting cool & pleasant. One letter from Maggie is all I have received from home in one month and a half. It was gratefully received I assure you. Give my love to all. Write soon & often & believe me ever

> *Your affectionate Son*
> *James D. Benton*
> *111th NY Vols*

*   *   *

Sept 25, 1863

Dear Parents,

I received a letter from Pa and Richardson just before we left Elkton but did not then have a chance to reply and have not had since until now and my facilities are at present very poor as we have to write on cracker boxes or whatever may come to hand.

Since we left Elkton we have been almost constantly on the march or picket duty and much exposed to the weather for several days being rainy and we had to wear our wet clothes as the wagon train was left behind. It has now been two weeks since I have had my pants off and no knowing how much longer it will be. We are in plain view of the Rebel pickets and have been since we have been here. When I finished the last page I thought I would stop

---

25 Frustrated by Meade's inability to finish off Lee's army above or below the Potomac River after the Gettysburg battle, Lincoln and the War Department pressed Meade to assume the offensive in Northern Virginia. The pressure, coupled with Lee's aggressive posture, would lead to the Bristoe Station and Mine Run campaigns that fall. Neither was successful and after the latter the Army of the Potomac would go into winter quarters.

until morning but it is rumored that we are to move soon so I thought I had better complete what I wanted to write.

I have been having a touch of my old complaint the Ague[26] for 8 or 10 days past brought on by the extraordinary exposure. I had a high fever last night and I have taken considerable Quinine[27] to-day so that I think shall break it up. Exposure to wet weather and sleeping on damp ground almost invariably brings on symptoms of it.

Of course you know where we are from the papers about as well as we do ourselves and we know but little of the whereabouts of the rest of the army. The cars run down to Mitchels Station about 6 miles below Culpepper Court House and Gen Meade's headquarters are supposed to be at the latter place. It is probable that the Rebs have no very large force on the other side of the river and that which is there is principally cavalry. It has been a terrible hard march since we left Elkton and many men have been made sick by the hard work & bad weather. We lay within a mile or mile & a half of the Rapidan [River] just at the end of Cedar Mountain[28] sometimes called Slaughter Mountain.

The Paymaster is here and we expect our Greenbacks soon, will get them in the morning I think. Those from our vicinity in the Regt. are well as usual. John Stoddard of Ira died the other day of fever and a Thoracic complication. I hear once a week from Maggie generally and am glad to hear

26 Ague is the least severe, but the most characteristic form of malarial disease. It is marked by four well-defined stages during each outburst. The first stage is the cold, or chill. The second is the hot stage, during which the sufferer's temperature can rise as high as 105 or 106 Fahrenheit, and is usually accompanied by pain and suffering in the head and back and vomiting. The third is the sweating stage, during which the high temperature and most of the pain subsides, leaving the patient weak and exhausted. The final stage is the intermission, or a period of no fever or any severe symptoms. This stage continues until the next "fit," which may occur within the next 24 to 72 hours. Ague can last for two and as long as three weeks.

27 Quinine, a bitter crystalline compound found in Cinchona bark, was used to treat malarial diseases. Side effects could include giddiness, deafness, ringing in the ears, and nausea. Large doses may be a source of danger by the direct sedative action of the drug on the nervous and circulatory systems.

28 Cedar Mountain was witness to a sizable battle on August 9, 1862 between troops led by Confederate Major General Thomas "Stonewall" Jackson and Union Major General Nathaniel P. Banks. The sharp fight is often considered the opening salvo of the Second Bull Run (Manassas) campaign fought at the end of that month. For a good tactical history of this fight, see Robert K. Krick, *Stonewall Jackson at Cedar Mountain* (Chapel Hill, 2002).

of her and Jessies good health. But I must stop as it is late. I hope to hear from you soon. Give my love to all.

> *Yours Affectionatly*
> *James D. Benton*
> *111th NY Vols*
> *3d Brigade 3d Division 2nd Army corps*
> *Army of the Potomac*
> *Washington D.C*

I dont like to send letters without stamps but we cant get them. I have sent for some. I enclose a curiosity called Rattle Snake weed, from the noise it makes.

* * *

> *Hd. Qurs. 111th N.Y.V.*
> *near Auburn Va.*
> *Oct. 21, 1863*

Dear Father,

I know you must think that I have neglected you in my correspondence lately but it has been unavoidable for a long time. We have been constantly on the march and it was impossible for me to write hardly any and not half the time we have been able to send or receive any mail. Well now for our situation.

We are about two miles south of Gainesville, which you will see is about west of Centreville Va. and also about six miles from Warrenton and near a village consisting of one house called Auburn. On the 14th we had a fight with some cavalry near here and killed and captured many of them, among whom (killed) was the celebrated Col. [Thomas] Ruffin[29] of North Carolina.

---

29 Colonel Thomas Ruffin was mortally wounded at the Battle of Auburn, Virginia, on October 13-14, 1863. He commanded the 1st North Carolina Cavalry Regiment in a charge against a line of infantry. The fight came about when Maj. Gen. Jeb Stuart's cavalry captured supply wagons and ran into the rear guard of the Union III Corps near Warrenton.

I will give you an outline of our march, starting from the Rapidan we went to Culpepper then to Rapahannock Station then to Bealton then to Liberty then to Catletts[30] *delaying long enough to lick the cavalry near here. Up the Rail Road to Bristow Station where the fight occurred at about 4 o'clock until dark. At about 9 o'clock we moved away without any noise and marched all night and got across Bull Run south of Centreville about 4 o'clock in the morning. We laid over until the 17th went to Bristow and then back to within a mile of Gainsville then down south about 9 miles where we have laid since yesterday the 20th. We have had very hard marching and but very little to eat and a chew of tobacco among the boys was worth 5 cents. The report now is that the Rebs have gone back across the Rappahannock, which from appearances is very probable.*

The 2nd Corps had a severe fight on the 14th at Bristow Station in which our division was engaged and the musketry was more severe than anytime at Gettysburg but the artillery was little used. Once in awhile a shell would fly over my head but the bullets whizzed much closer and very frequent. We were on one side of the Rail Road and the Rebels on the other and both ran to gain it our boys got to it first and once behind the bush they were comparatively safe and laid the Rebels thick upon the ground in front until they retreated back to the woods. We took 450 prisoners and six abandoned Rebel guns.

The reporters dont tell the truth about this battle. It lasted about 3 hours stopping at dark and at about 9 o'clock it was very dark and we moved along up the Rail Road marching all night and crossing Bull Run near Centreville about 4 o'clock AM and laid down in the mud and rain to get a little sleep. The Rebs are said to have retreated at the same time the wagon train was what they wanted and it was a mutual surprise to both armies. But we flaxed them nicely and Genl. Hill received a very sudden check in his purposes.[31]

---

30 A former stop along the strategically vital Orange and Alexandria Railroad, which was the target of many raids during the war.

31 Ambrose Powell Hill was promoted to lead the newly formed Third Corps after the death of Thomas Jackson in May 1863. The battle of Bristoe Station, October 14, 1863, resulted when Hill's vanguard came upon a large body of retreating Union troops. The aggressive Hill attacked without proper reconnaissance and men from the Union II Corps, most from behind an embankment on the Orange & Alexandria Railroad, tore apart two Rebel brigades and captured an artillery battery. This period of the war has been mostly overlooked. See Bill Backus and Rob Orrison, *A Want of Vigilance: The Bristoe Station Campaign, October 9–19, 1863* (Savas Beatie, 2015), part of the Emerging Civil War series. Hill was killed during the final day of the Petersburg Campaign on April 2, 1865.

I see I have finished my paper and must stop. My conveniences for writing is a seat on the ground and the light of a rail fire so if it is not very legible you must attribute it to that. My health is quite good at present and the Ague does not trouble me as much lately. The mail is going out and I must stop. Give my love to all. Let me hear from you as soon as possible. Sometimes I cant write because we dont stay long enough in one place but I think we will stay here a day or two.

Your Affectionate Son
J D Benton

*   *   *

Head Quarters
111th N.Y.V.
Oct. 23, 1863

Dear Father,

I had just written you a letter the day before I received yours but you make inquiries not contained in it and to reply to those I write to-day again.

In my last [letter] I told you what we had done in a military point of view which it is not necessary for me to reiterate. My health is I think improving for I have not been well since we moved from Elkton six weeks since. The chief difficulty being the Ague for which this country is famous. All the types of fever we have here commence in this way soon becoming continued, fever accompanied with irritation of the bowels.

Our fare, the thing which concerns us most is of quite an indifferent kind but wholesome and I can assure you very plain. On the march we are many times in straightened circumstances in this respect for we may not see the supply train for a week and the [indecipherable word] are ordered away. We get hungry many times. We get hardtack[32] or pilot bread at 5 cents per pound fresh beef at 10 cents, occasionally potatoes most always coffee and sugar.

---

32 Hardtack is a plain flour and water biscuit about three inches square and half an inch thick, baked brick-hard. The bread was often wormy, and so hard it broke teeth. Soldiers on both sides often made jokes about how difficult it was to consume.

This of course we have to carry and cook ourselves and we cant have much variety. Sometimes we fry our hardtack in pork and sometimes stew it with the same after soaking it in cold water. It may be boiled 24 hours in water and it will only be the tougher but cold water will soften it.

You ask if I am ever homesick and want to leave the service. I answer once in awhile but very seldom although I should like to see you all very much. I can make more here than anywhere else and where our chances are the best we ought to stay.

You ask about the sick and how many we have, I reply not any as soon as a man is taken sick he is immediately sent away unless it be with some slight disorder from which he will recover in a few days. It would be impossible to take any care of sick men here having no hospital regimental or otherwise besides if a fight occurs it would not do to have the ambulances filled up with sick and be compelled to leave the wounded on the field to be made prisoners. It would do either to carry them around the country as we have to march so often we have just arrived in our present camp having moved this morning from where I last wrote you.

We now lay on the R.R. between Warrenton and Warrenton Junction. The Rebels are said to have gone back across the Rappahannock. The object of the movement of our army up and back it is impossible to fathom but in my opinion is that its object is to deceive the enemy and that we will all soon go back to the defenses of Washington and all of this army except what is necessary for its defenses will be sent to Chattanooga [Tennessee] and join the Army of the Cumberland. This is all supposition and that is all it is worth.

I have written quite a lengthy letter and it must suffice for now. May it find you all in good health and spirits. My love to Ma and all the rest. I received a letter from Laura yesterday she writes finely. Let me hear from you soon.

Your Affectionate Son
James D. Benton

*   *   *

Seminary Hospital
Georgetown D.C.
Nov. 16, 1863

Dear Father,

It has been some time since I wrote you last and I thought I would write what I could to-night as you might think it strange in not hearing from me sooner. You probably know from my letters to Maggie where I am.

It is a week yesterday since I came into the hospital here and my health has greatly improved during that time. When I came I was better than I had been previously and the change from the ground to a good bed and comfortable room did me much good. My disease was the same as I had been troubled with most of the fall viz intermittent fever with diarrhea which latter I had about two months and I was very fearful that it would become chronic and be very difficult to get rid of but I am glad to say that I am better in this respect [but] still not wholly free from it. The two difficulties together produced a degree of debility that made it impossible for me to do anything and the heavy marching we had to do during that time about used me up. My fever has stopped but I am very weak and slight exertion starts the sweat. I am in hopes that I may get a leave of absence for a short time at least I am going to try it. I have good accommodations in all respects and good care. This hospital is exclusively for officers, the only one in the city I believe of the kind. It is full of sick and wounded but only one or two dangerously so.

The most trouble I have is that I get lonesome lying here all the time but during the coming week I am going to get out around the city and try to shake myself up a little. The weather here is splendid and quite warm. During last week the streets were very dusty but a rain storm has stopped that and it is cool at night but very pleasant in the daytime. I suppose you begin to think about sleighing at home.

There does not appear to be any army news at present. I am told that army headquarters are at Brandy Station doubtless waiting for the completion of the Rail Road which is nearly done. I am inclined to think that there will be another fight before a great while in Virginia. And I am confident that the cry "On to Richmond" never could be obeyed any easier than at this time. It would bring on a severe engagement but I think it would be more decisive than any hitherto.

I must stop now. My love to all and I hope to hear from you soon.

Your Affectionate Son,
James D. Benton

*   *   *

Head Quarters 111th
Dec. 22nd 1863

Dear Parents,

I take the first good opportunity to write not only to let you know that the present is favorable but also to apprise you of the past movements of the army its purposes and the causes, of its failure as far as the last short campaign is concerned.

I found an article in the New York Times, which is as far as I can learn a correct description of the movement. I have talked with many officers and they described the scene before the expected charge on the Rebel works as a very affecting one as the chances of a mans coming out alive were as one in ten. There they stood in easy musket shot of the enemy having thrown off knapsacks and every encumbrance to double quick, officers bidding each other good bye, making their wills, and leaving tokens of affection for those at home. But it was delayed and we all admire Genl. Warren[33] for his conduct when he said to Meade, "I will obey the order but there will be no 2nd Corps left" and when Meade was fully aware of the situation he approved his course in every particular. A careful reading of the piece will give you a good

---

33 New York native Gouverneur Kemble Warren graduated from West Point in 1850 second in his class. From graduation until the Civil War he served in the topographical engineers. Warren commanded a brigade at Second Bull Run and Antietam, and was promoted to brigadier general on September 26, 1862, and major general on August 8, 1863. While serving as the Army of the Potomac's chief engineer, Warren identified the importance of Little Round Top on July 2, 1863, and organized its initial defense. He temporarily led Hancock's II Corps from August 1863 until March 1864, when he was assigned to head the V Corps when the Army of the Potomac was reshuffled for the Overland Campaign. Warren was relieved of his command during the Five Forks battle on April 1 by Philip Sheridan, and spent the remainder of his life trying to clear his name.

idea of the abandonment and the proposed plan of attack which had it not been for a blunder or two would have been disastrous to the enemy.[34]

Now for our present situation. Almost south of Brandy Station if you look at the map you will see a place by the name of Stephensburg, which like all Virginia towns looks larger on the map than anywhere else. We are located about a mile north-east of it on a high ridge of hills from which Culpepper and Slaughter [Cedar] Mountains can be plainly seen. I never saw a more beautiful prospect probably in consequence of its great extent and the long Blue Ridge in the distance.

We have good log huts put up and it looks as if a large body of men had gone into the woods in a new country and was about to build a city. Camps of all kinds can be seen as far as the eye can reach either way and all things denote winter quarters. But I must stop first saying that I am in good health and spirits. Let me hear from you soon.

Yours Affectionately,
James D Benton

P.S. Dr. Vosburgh has gone home on a sick leave and I of course am now the "great mogul" of the Medical Department of the Regt.

---

34 Dr. Benton is referring to the Mine Run Campaign (November 26 - December 2, 1863), when Meade crossed the Rapidan River to flank Lee's army and defeat it. An accidental meeting by parts of both armies at Payne's Farm on the 27th led to a bloody fight, buying Lee time to withdraw behind Mine Run creek, where he had established (and improved) a defensive position. Tasked with turning the Rebel flank, Warren conducted a march around Lee's right only to discover massive works he determined unassailable. Meade had ordered an army-wide assault at a given hour; Warren's impassioned plea convinced Meade to cancel it. Little has been written about this interesting campaign.

1864

Ulysses S. Grant's willingness to fight and his ability to win in the Western Theater impressed President Lincoln. Although often overlooked or even slighted by the likes of Major General Henry Halleck and others, Grant persisted, keeping large-scale goals in mind as he achieved one victory after another despite the difficulties and setback he encountered along the way. His was exactly the attitude Lincoln was seeking, and the president promoted Grant to lieutenant general, a rank not awarded since George Washington.[1] Lincoln also made Grant the commander of all the Union armies, and set upon his shoulders the responsibility of ultimate Union victory.

1 Ulysses S. Grant was born April 27, 1822 in Point Pleasant, Ohio, appointed to West Point in 1839, and graduated four years later 21st out of 39. He saw service during the Mexican War, but left the army thereafter to try a variety of trades, none of which proved successful. When the Civil War began, Grant was appointed colonel of the 21st Illinois and a few months later brigadier general. He began proving his worth in the field in February of 1862 when he captured Forts Henry and Donelson and was promoted to major general. Although surprised at Shiloh that April, Grant remained in place and beat back the enemy attack. After several failed attempts to capture Vicksburg, Mississippi, he launched a bold combined operations offensive that trapped the Rebels inside the city; they surrendered on July 4, 1863. After accepting Robert E. Lee's surrender at Appomattox on April 9, 1865, Grant was elected president in 1868. He served two terms, both marked by scandal and corruption. The heavy cigar smoker died from throat cancer on July 23, 1885 at Mount McGregor, New York, after finishing his memoirs. For a good new biography of Grant, see Ronald C. White, *American Ulysses: A Life of Ulysses S. Grant* (Random House, 2016).

Rather than remain in the nation's capital and direct the Union armies from there, Grant decided to take the field with General Meade's Army of the Potomac that spring of 1864 when it moved against General Lee's Army of Northern Virginia. Grant placed his favorite subordinate and friend Major General William Tecumseh Sherman in command of Union forces in the Western Theater.[2]

Grant was determined to prosecute the war to a successful conclusion, but in a different fashion than heretofore undertaken. Rather than allowing armies to operate mostly independently of one another, he decided to make several simultaneous advances from Virginia to Georgia to pin Confederate armies in position and thus not allow them to use their interior lines to reinforce one another. He also made it clear that the enemy armies were the main goal; he did not expect to fight a battle and retreat. Unlike every other Union commander thus far, Grant fully grasped the manpower advantage enjoyed by the North, and knew that if the armies in blue gripped their opponents and refused to let them go, regardless of a tactical loss, the South would be bled dry and have no choice but to eventually surrender.

The newly minted lieutenant general was also willing to fight something closer to "total war" by allowing his armies to live off the land, burn Southern barns and crops, and destroy railroads and telegraph lines. He intended to cripple the Confederacy by killing its soldiers and weaken the morale of those at home. Grant's Overland Campaign and Sherman's Atlanta Campaign both opened in early May.

*   *   *

---

2 William Tecumseh Sherman (born February 8, 1820 in Lancaster, Ohio), graduated West Point in 1840, and spent most of his Civil War career in the Western Theater. He led a division at Shiloh, saw extensive action under Grant (though his overall performance was rather mixed), set out for Atlanta in May 1864, which he captured that September. Sherman burned the city and marched to the sea late that fall, captured Savannah at the end of 1864, and thrust north in early 1865 into the Carolinas, where he accepted Joe Johnston's surrender in late April. The latest major study of the man is James Lee McDonough, *William Tecumseh Sherman: In the Service of My Country. A Life* (W. W. Norton & Co., 2017). A deep objective study of the general's military service, however, has yet to be written.

The U.S. Christian Commission[3] sends this as the soldier's messenger to his home. Let it hasten to those who wait for tidings.

Head Quarters 111th NYV
Feb. 8, 1864

Dear Parents,

I have time only to write a very few lines but thought that I would do so that I might hear from you. Do you realize that I have not had a letter from my father and mother since I left home[?]. I cant understand why it is but it is so and I am sorry that it is so for I would very much like to hear from you.

We, as you will see by the papers, have been engaged in a fight again although we have not suffered very much.[4] Only two being wounded seriously neither of whom belonged in our neighborhood. Several were slightly hurt but our regiment was on the whole very fortunate. The number of killed and wounded in the Division will number about two hundred in all.

Our Division left camp on Saturday morning the 6th and went down to the Rapidan River reaching it at Mortons Ford a distance of about three miles. They drove in the pickets of the enemy, capturing about thirty [men] and crossed the river under an artillery fire. The water was up to the armpits of the soldiers. This was on Saturday and as I said before, the fight was short and in the night our Division was withdrawn to this side of the river and lay down on the ground in their wet clothes they stayed there all day Sunday and at night returned to camp. The object was to ascertain the position and force of the enemy but I am sorry it cost so much perhaps it is all for the best.

---

3   The United States Christian Commission was instituted in November of 1861. Its goal was to promote the spiritual and temporal welfare of the soldiers. The commission supplied periodicals, books, and religious tracts, such as bibles.

4   The Battle of Morton's Ford (February 6-7, 1864). Elements of the Army of the Potomac forced three crossings of the Rapidan River on February 6 in an effort to distract Southern attention from a mixed arms (cavalry and infantry) raid up the Virginia peninsula on Richmond. Part of the II Corps crossed at Morton's Ford, the I Corps at Raccoon Ford, and Union cavalry at Robertson's Ford. Elements from the Confederate Second Corps under Richard S. Ewell resisted the crossings, with the most severe fighting coming at Morton's. The attacks ended on the 7th and the Union forces withdrew that night. The effort was for nothing because no troops were dispatched from Richmond, and no raid was made against the city. Losses totaled 262 Union and about 60 Rebels killed and wounded.

Tell Maggie that Lieut[enant] Shields, one of Genl Hays aids was wounded through the chest near the heart and probably will die. She knows him I guess.

Our regiment is truly the fighting Regt. of our state and none consists of braver or better men and officers and none have done better service than it. Our Corps is to be recruited up to 50,000 men and will be assigned to a special duty in the spring, which special duty undoubtedly will be to go down on the Peninsula and take Richmond acting in concert of course with other portions of the army.

But I must stop for it is late and I am quite tired as I have just come in from picket. So I will [go] to bed. I have looked anxiously for letters from you and have written still I get none and I thought I would write once more. Give my love to all and let me hear from you as soon as possible.

Yours Affectionately
James D. Benton
Asst. Surg, 111th N.Y.V.[5]

*   *   *

Camp of the 111th N.Y.V.
March 6, 1864

Dear Parents,

I have already too long delayed replying to your letter but I will not weary you with the infinite excuses so often used by letter writers and let it suffice to say that I have not written before and am now at it.

We continue in the same camp [Brandy Station] that we have occupied all winter and will doubtless not leave it until active operations begin in the spring although we are constantly harassed by camp rumors that we are going to move every two or three days.

You seem to be somewhat astonished that the doctors have to do picket duty and inquire why it is. I do not mean to have you to imply that we do the duty of a solider on the picket line by any means but that every day a surgeon

5   In March 1864, the 111th became part of the 3rd Brigade, 1st Division, II Corps.

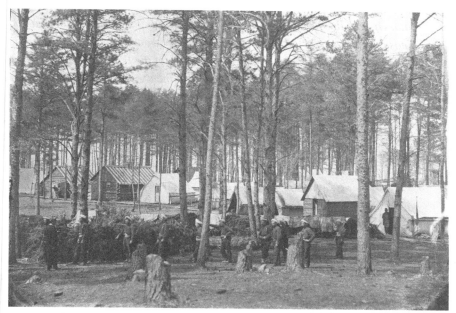

Brandy Station, Virginia, the camp of the Army of the Potomac, April 1864. *LOC*

is sent out in charge of the picket of each Division and stays until relieved by his successor on the succeeding day. The object of this is that in case of accident or attack by the enemy he can be at hand or in case of sickness he can send in to camp with a written excuse for the person who may be ill. The authority of a surgeon over sick men is supreme and when either officer or man is excused from duty by them no one however high in military authority can with safety interfere with it.

Of course you have seen an account of the "grand raid" of [Judson] Kilpatrick[6] into Dixie and the excitement which he threw the Confederates

6   Dr. Benton is referencing the Kilpatrick-Dahlgren Raid (February 28–March 3, 1864), a bold effort by Judson Kilpatrick's Union cavalry to strike the Rebel capital at Richmond and free prisoners held there. The effort was a complete fiasco. Kilpatrick's main column halted at the city's defenses and later abandoned the effort, while a smaller supporting column under Col. Ulric Dahlgren, the young son of Admiral John Dahlgren, was ambushed and routed (and Dahlgren killed). Handwritten orders found on his corpse (later published in Richmond) included plans to burn the city and kill President Jefferson Davis and his cabinet. It appears they were genuine, but who wrote them remains unknown. Several books and magazines cover this topic, including Stephen W. Sears, *Controversies and Commanders: Dispatches from the Army of the Potomac* (Houghton Mifflin, 2001).

into. His cavalry force all or nearly all lays within half a mile of our camp. Those which went on the raid are in Genl Butler's department[7] and will soon be back here. I send you with this letter a copy of the Washington Chronicle with quite an extended account of his bold maneuvers.

The spring campaign will soon be upon us and in my opinion we have never seen any fighting which will equal what is coming. It will be the climax of desperation. We are all satisfied that however short the campaign may be that its battles will be fought to the bitter end and mercy will be a scarce article.

But I must soon stop. I have not had a letter from Maggie for a long time and am much surprised that she dont write oftener lately. In fact I think I have been neglected by all. I received and answered a letter from ARB a few days since all were well there in Indiana.

My love to all and in the hope to hear from you all soon I remain,

Yours Affectionately
James D. Benton

*   *   *

Dr. Benton's words proved prescient. Two months before the opening of the spring campaign, he had written his father, "we have never seen any fighting which will equal what is coming. It will be the climax of desperation." His next nine letters were written during the Petersburg siege (June 15, 1864 – April 2, 1865), the longest campaign of the Civil War.

About 25 miles south of Richmond, Petersburg was a major logistical and manufacturing hub with railroads radiating north to Richmond and south to connect with other parts of the crumbling Confederacy. Without Petersburg, Richmond would fall and Lee's army could not be supplied.

In order to reach Petersburg, Grant and Meade led the Army of the Potomac through the Overland Campaign, a bloody series of combats beginning with the Wilderness in early May through Spotsylvania, the North Anna fighting, Cold Harbor, and the crossing of the James River in mid-June. The extremely heavy losses (suffered by both armies), and the nearly

---

7 Maj. Gen. Benjamin Butler operated on the peninsula in command of the Army of the James.

James's June 5, 1864, letter home. *Author*

relentless fighting did not put off Grant, who knew he was seriously weakening the Confederacy's ability to remain in the field.

The siege of Petersburg began in mid-June 1864 after a series of bungled Union attacks that should have captured the lightly defended city failed.

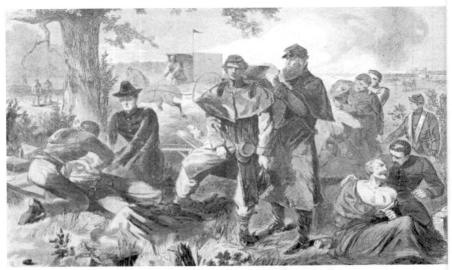

"The Surgeon at Work in the Rear During an Engagement" by Winslow Homer.
Harper's Weekly

Once Lee's army rushed south of the James River and into defenses, however, it was no longer possible to quickly take the vital rail and production center. Grant settled into a methodical siege, long lines of trenches sprang up, and both Richmond and Petersburg became locked into a siege-style combat that would not end until April 1865.

*   *   *

June 5, 1864

Dear Parents

I received Pa's letter dated May 26 last night and hasten to reply although there is much to write about I am not sure that I can make out much of a letter and you must bear with me if it is not very interesting.

I rejoined the regiment several days since from Fredericksburg, [Virginia] and since I returned the fighting has been every day continuous. We are now on the road leading to New Bridge and about two miles from the Chickahominy River with lots of Johnnie's between but the utmost confidence prevails that we can go through with the journey we have

The end of James's letter home dated June 5, 1864, with his signature. *Author*

undertaken. Richmond is about 10 miles from our front but the road was very succinctly described to me by one of our soldiers who said that it "was a good ways from home, up hill, and d——d sandy."

All the letters which came to the Regt for me were sent to Fredericksburg and the mail communication being given up they probably are in Washington but will eventually come on to me so you see I have had only two letters since I left home one from Maggie and yours.

You wish to know if I wish to sell the place at Ira. I do and think best to dispose of it for eleven hundred or [what] can be got. I probably shall never locate there again.

You wish to have me give you some of the incidents of the battles but I must say that it is almost impossible for me to do so for my time has been so much occupied with the care of the wounded that very little of my attention could be given to the details of military movements. All we know is that

[Ulysses Simpson] Grant is master of the situation and that he proposes to fight it out on this line if it takes all summer.[8]

It is said that Genls. [John] Pope & [David] Hunter have landed at White House [landing on the James River] and are on the way. We have now the 2nd-5th-6th-9th-10th-18th Corps here and a many thousand men not yet organized into any Corps so you see we have men enough and we have 15 or 20 acres of artillery that have not yet fired a shot.

When we see this army we cant form any conception of its strength. It is admirably organized and has the utmost confidence in its commanders. They are in telegraph communication with each other and Genl. Grant. Probably you wonder how this can be done so easily and I will tell you. The wire used is covered with Gutta Percha and is wound around windlasses and carried in wagons. When they want to put up a telegraph they take out a windlass full of wire and fasten it by a saddle to a mules back and get the mule under motion. The wire is unwound and they lay it up on the limbs of trees on poles or even on the ground from any part of the army necessary to any other part.

We carry mortars in wagons which shell the Rebels in style. We have had hard work for the past month, hard tack and pork is about all we get (fresh beef occasionally) and until I joined the Regt. I had not changed my clothes in three weeks sleeping in all of them most of the time.

But I have about finished my sheet and must stop for the present. I suppose you had heard of Wallace Fink being killed his bro[ther] Manning was wounded trying to get away his body.[9]

I hope to hear from you very soon again. Good Bye.

Your son,

J.D. Benton

---

8   Dr. Benton is quoting a sentence from Grant's letter to Secretary of War Stanton on May 11 during the early days of the Spotsylvania campaign, when he wrote "I propose to fight it out on this line if it takes all summer."

9   Private Wallace Fink, Company H, was killed (and his brother Manning wounded) outside Richmond in the fighting at Bethesda Church, Virginia.

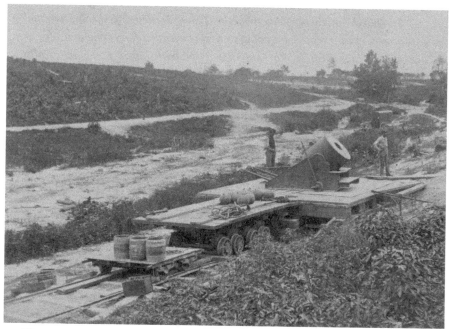

The "Dictator," a 13-inch mortar outside Petersburg, Virginia. Dr. Benton would have heard its deep-throated roar as it lobbed its heavy shells into the Rebel lines. *LOC*

P.S. I can cheerfully say for the Sanitary Commission that it is saving thousands and thousands of lives. J.D.B. [10]

*   *   *

Head Quarters 111th N.Y.V. [11]
July 22nd 1864

Dear Parents,

---

10 The Sanitary Commission was a private relief agency created by Congress on June 18, 1861, to offer support to sick and wounded Union soldiers. It enlisted the help of thousands of individuals, raised millions of dollars, and did extraordinary work across the entire North.

11 That June, the 111th New York was transferred to the Consolidated Brigade, 1st Division, II Corps, where it would remain until November 1864.

I do not distinctly remember whether I have written since I received your last or not, at all events I am going to write because I have time to do so.

To-day has been remarkably quiet on both sides. Once in awhile however we hear a heavy gun booming away at some object over towards Petersburg and then in a short time it receives a reply from our neighbor on the opposite side. We have changed our location a little since I wrote you last at that time we lay almost on the extreme left of the army but on Tuesday night last we had orders to be in readiness to march at a moments notice and we had not long to wait. We marched still farther to the left and rested until dark on Wednesday night when we marched down near the Weldon Rail Road in order to protect the rear of some cavalry while destroying the road we returned the same night before daylight and after a short rest marched to the place where we now lay which is in the rear of the 9th Corps and about a mile and a half from the city of Petersburg.

Some of the heavy guns are a short distance from us and from the hill in front we can see almost on to the city. I can sit in the door of my tent and see the shells explode in the air and in the night the long trail of the mortar shells go through the air like comets on a fandango. A person is much safer to stand from under.

We have not been engaged with the enemy since I wrote you and when we reached our present camp orders were given to put up tents and lay out streets in regular camp. There is a rumor to-day that Grant has notified the Johnnies that Petersburg is in a state of siege and advised them to remove the women and children for safety. Whether this is true or not I do not know, but I do know that there are preparations on for which will astonish the Rebels before long.[12]

The health of the Regt. is usually good the principle difficulty being diarrhea. I shall be obliged to postpone the rest of the letter until tomorrow in consequence of darkness.

12 Dr. Benton may have been referring to the tunneling efforts being made on a different part of the line by Pennsylvania soldiers with coal mining experience. The tunnel they dug under the Confederate lines was packed with explosives and detonated early on the morning of July 30, 1864, just a little more than a week after he penned this letter. The subsequent "Battle of the Crater" began well for Union armies, but ended in a bloody fiasco when thousands of African-American troops were trapped in the crater left by the blast and slaughtered there.

22d: There is nothing new in the way of news since yesterday. The batteries created a monstrous amount of noise last night throwing shells to & fro. Some of these big guns make things shake considerably. The weather has moderated a great deal in the past few days as far as heat is concerned and now a good fresh breeze is blowing. Two or three days since we had a good shower of rain and followed by this cool wind makes Virginia life much more endurable than heretofore. I see by the papers that a draft is pending and I am glad that the commutation clause is so disposed of that the Gov[ernmen]t will get men and not money. I do not want either of my brothers to be drafted of course but it is the only way to raise men and the men must be had. The life of an officer is in all respects hard enough and a private soldier has much more to endure.

To-day is my twenty seventh birth-day and it is lacks not quite a month of two years that I have been in the service. What a long tedious two years it has been no one but myself can imagine.

But I must close my letter for my sheet is about full. I trust you will write very often and tell me all the home news. My love to all at home.

As Ever Your Affectionate Son,
James D. Benton

*   *   *

Head Quarters 111th N.Y.V.
Aug 2nd 1864

Dear Father,

I considered myself doubly fortunate this morning in getting letters from you and Maggie at the same time.

Since I wrote you last we have been on a raid as the papers have doubtless already informed you. On the afternoon of Wednesday the 27th, the 2nd Corps was ordered to move and got under motion about sunset, destination to us as usual unknown. The general impression was that we were to go to Washington to repel the invasion there and as the head of the column pointed towards City Point the idea gained credence and all were full of joy at the prospect of going into the defenses of the Capital. But all our fond anticipations were doomed to be crushed for on nearing City Point we turned sharp to the left through a circuitous route to the Appomattox River, crossing a long pontoon bridge about 10 o'clock into the dominions of [General Benjamin] "Beast Butler."

After a short rest we marched on our general course being towards the James River and we reached it at about 3 o'clock in the morning and rested for a short time on Jones's neck and crossed on a pontoon covered with hay and pine boughs to muffle the sound. We formed a line of battle at nearly right angles to the river and behind a narrow strip of magnificent oaks and waited for day. At about 7 o'clock the order to "fall in" was given [and] a Brigade of each division was deployed as skirmishers and the balance formed in line of battle and advanced to the further edge of a woods. Beyond was an open field and woods on the opposite side the main line now advanced about half way across the open space and the skirmish line pushed forward towards the Rebs who lay in the timber beyond and it was done so dexterously that the Johnnies had to fall back leaving in our hands four twenty pound rifled parrot guns of the best sort. We also captured several prisoners. The cavalry and infantry were maneuvering around all day Thursday and Friday to give the impression of [a] large force. The cavalry also took about 100 prisoners.

Friday night we all slid and Saturday morning found us again in front of Petersburg and the dance began at once. By this movement a large part of Lee's army had gone to the defence of Richmond and when we got back were there yet.[13] The first we know up goes a Rebel fort and a Regt of Rebs and sixteen guns fifty feet into the air and a hundred and twenty guns open the bombardment of Petersburg. I cant give any description of the fuss on paper and I dont know as I could by words, but I imagine the infernal regions may bear somewhat of a resemblance. An assault was made and we were partially successful and for a time held their line but it was finally relinquished and we remain as we were before. A great blunder has been committed by somebody

---

13 The purpose of the march earlier described by Dr. Benton was to convince General Lee that a main effort would be made against Richmond in the hope he would weaken his Petersburg defenses to bolster those north of the James River in preparation for the detonation of the Petersburg mine on July 30, 1864.

and we hear an investigation is to be had but that will not restore the limbs and lives of 3 or 4000 that fell that day.[14]

The fault is generally attributed to subordinate commanders and the skill manifested by Grant, Meade, and [Winfield Scott] Hancock[15] in executing the movement absolves them from all blame. There is no question that at least one half of the force in Petersburg doublequicked it for the other side of the James River to repel what they considered a formidable force attacking Richmond and we have lost a golden opportunity which I am fearful we shall not meet with again. The first reports of the Petersburg affair were of great success but we were doomed to disappointment in the after part of the engagement. We trust some other course may disclose itself to Grant to drive them from this point.

Our news from Atlanta is good and encourages us.[16] It is rumored that our two divisions are going to the defense of Washington. How true it is we do not know but there are some indications of it. The rumor puts Hancock in command of that Department. We know he was offered that command before but would not accept unless he could take his corps certainly nothing could be more acceptable to us than that arrangement.

The paymasters are around and we expect our money soon, we are all much in need of it. The weather for the past week has been cooler and more comfortable than for a long time past with occasional showers of rain of short duration however.

I was grieved to hear of the death of Bassett and wish to hear the particulars in your next [letter]. There is no extraordinary amount of sickness here except diarrhoea, which is always prevalent in the army more or less.

But I must close as I have made out quite a sizeable letter considering the heat and the flies which annoy us terribly. Let me hear from you as soon

14 For a good study on the Crater battle, see Earl J. Hess, *Into the Crater: The Mine Attack at Petersburg* (Columbia, 2010).

15 Winfield Scott Hancock, a West Point graduate of the Class of 1844, was the commander of the II Corps in the Army of the Potomac.

16 By this time, Sherman's armies had driven deep into Georgia and were investing Atlanta. The Confederate commander of the opposing Army of Tennessee, Gen. Joseph E. Johnston, had been replaced by Gen. John B. Hood, whose attacks against the larger Union force had been rebuffed at Peach Tree Creek (July 20), Battle of Atlanta (July 22), and Ezra Church (July 28).

as possible and give me all the news for home matters are of much interest to me. I saw Dr. W[illia]m. Root the other day they are in this neighborhood now and are in the 19th Corps. My love to all as ever.

Your Affectionate Son
James D. Benton

*   *   *

Head Quarters
111th N.Y.V.
Sept 15th 1864
Dear Parents,

It is some time since I have had any letters from home and I waited in daily expectation of one until now so I concluded I would write and call your attention to the fact. I am truly in want of news and I get quite lonesome if I dont hear from you more frequently.

I had a good letter from Laura last night and have just replied to it she tells me considerable news especially as to who had enlisted and how she was getting along. I see by the papers that New York will not suffer much from the draft and it is a source of gratification to those in the field to know they are not forgotten by the loyal population of the north and it is the general impression that Grant will close this thing up before a great while.

I do not doubt that the Rebels expect much from political results this fall and neither do I doubt that their disappointment will be certain and very bitter. In my mind the election of Abraham [Lincoln] is as sure as it can be and in the Union army he will find his strongest support. I hope I may have a chance to cast my vote for him. He was the first President I ever voted for and if he is the last the Union ever has he will be my choice. I know that he is honest and I do not want to barter him away for one of doubtful honesty. I wonder how the Democratic Peace Convention fancies [General] McClellan's acceptance of the nomination. His letter of acceptance is the wet blanket to cool the fever of their platform. Politics go rather slow here in the army and very little excitement exists about the coming election. Grant is to make all the peace we will have very soon.[17]

We are still at Petersburg and operations are going on as usual. Picket firing and cannonading are going on kept up most of the time with occasional fits and starts. The way Grant celebrated the fall of Atlanta was a caution. It was ahead of all the pyrotechnic displays I ever witnessed and more grandly terrible than the whole Revolutionary War and all the independence days from that time to this. If the John Henry's over the line were not astonished they must be very dull of comprehension. I was where I had a fair sight although none too far away to be agreeable and it was a majestic sight. By Grants order every gun and mortar shells sailing through the air with their peculiar sound at 12 o'clock at night was sublimely grand and a good deal of the hideous mixed.

I am as well as usual and try to enjoy myself as much as possible. I sent $300 to Pa Rich sometime since and as I have not heard a word about its reception I am naturally anxious to know of its safe arrival do you know anything of it?

I have nearly exhausted my sheet and must close up. Give my love to all at home and let me hear from you as soon as possible. I remain as ever.

Your Affectionate Son
James D Benton

*   *   *

Head Quarters
111th N.Y.V.
Sept 21st 1864

Dear Parents,

17 Many in the Confederacy pinned their hopes on Abraham Lincoln losing the November 1864 presidential election, but as Dr. Benton speculated, they would be disappointed. Lincoln ran under the National Union banner against his former top Civil War general and Democratic candidate George B. McClellan, who ran as the "peace candidate," though he did not personally believe in his party's platform. Once Atlanta fell in early September, and major Union victories were achieved in the Shenandoah Valley, the outcome was all-but assured.

I received a letter from Pa last night and was very glad to hear from home for it had been some time since I had had any letter. I was glad to learn that the money I had sent was safe. I do not exactly like the idea of investing it in county bonds and [would] much rather have it in the Government 7.30 which I consider much more desirable. Uncle Sam is a very safe Paymaster and [I] prefer him to any other.

We have just received the news of Sheridan's success in the [Shenandoah] Valley.[18] It came by telegraph and communication to the army by which it was received with great cheering and enthusiasm insomuch that Ulysses gave the enemy a salute at daylight this morning similar to the one after the fall of Atlanta.

We are still near the same spot that we have been in so long only we are a little nearer the Johnnies than before and act as a reserve to the Third Division of our Corps which lies in front. The gray chaps are in plain sight a few steps from our camp and their bullets sometimes visit us but we have a good barricade in front of our tents, which keeps off all the intruders of small size. What the big ones might do I do not know.

The weather is delightful and we get watermelons, apples, and peaches, which we find of great advantage to us in a sanitary point of view. I never felt so well in a long time as for the past month. It is becoming cooler and the leaves in the woods are getting a little yellow from age. It is wonderful to see how fast the army is filling up by returning convalescents and recruits. Every train from City Point brings up a load and they are distributed to their various regiments.

Dr. John Guffin is camped close to me and tells me much about my former Indiana acquaintances. I was very glad to see him indeed. The Rebels are very quiet and there was a rumor the other day that they had removed most of their heavy guns away from this position but it is not authentic and I doubt the truth of the rumor.

---

18 Major General Philip Sheridan (West Point Class of 1853) served with Grant in the Western Theater. His successes there resulted in Grant promoting him to lead the cavalry of the Army of the Potomac in 1864. In July of 1864 Sheridan was placed in command of the VI and XIX corps, three divisions of cavalry, and artillery. He was ordered to destroy everything in the Shenandoah Valley that could be used to support the Confederacy. To counter the move, Lee dispatched a large portion of his own army to reinforce the small Confederate force operating there, all under the command of Lt. Gen. Jubal Early. A series of high profile battles unfolded, including the stunning Union victory at Third Winchester on September 19, which is the success to which Dr. Benton refers.

We have received our printed votes and will favor Father Abraham by a large majority. I wrote you a day or so since and so I will not extend this one any further at present. I am as ever.

Your Affectionate Son
James D Benton

*   *   ***

Sept 27th 1864

Dear Parents,

I have just finished a long letter to Maggie and as I thought I might kill "two birds with one stone" I will write you also.

I am somewhat differently situated now than when I last wrote. I am now detailed as one of the hospital staff at our Division hospital and hold the office of Secretary and Recorder, which is a very pleasant and easy position. My duties are to see that the books, records, and papers are properly kept, the reports correctly and promptly made out and forwarded and attend to the admission of patients. The labor is mostly performed by a clerk and it is my business to see that it is done and done properly. I like it more than anything else for the reason that I have good quarters and more comfortable accommodations than I could have with the Regiment.

Our Brigade is now in the front of entrenchments and behind good breastworks eight feet high and ten [feet] thick at the top. They also have bomb proofs constructed as a defence against mortar shells which come more directly down. Of course you are all rejoiced at the cheering prospect of war matters which look so bright lately. The fact is that old Mr. Grant is after them with a sharp stick and if I am not much mistaken you will soon hear of a fracas in this region. I think [Gen. William] Sherman and Sheridan's operations have a greater bearing on our immediate situation here than is generally supposed.

There has been quite a change in the position of the forces here within the past few days. Our corps occupies the place of the 9th and 10th Corps, which leaves them a liberty for other operations. Ours and the 5th Corps hold the entire line south of the Appomattox [River] and if you dont see one of Grants tricks in a few days I am much mistaken. Everything looks bright as far as the war is concerned and Mr. Lee will soon be compelled to "git up and git." The probability Grant is waiting for him to send reinforcements to [Jubal] Early and as soon as he does down comes Petersburg with a rush.

Every soldier is worth ten percent more in consequence of the success in the Valley and in Georgia. Have you seen Sherman's letter to the Mayor of Atlanta in answer to one praying for a revocation of his order compelling the citizens to leave? It is pronounced to be the ablest thing from any General. I never read anything so concise and to the purpose.[19]

We receive the news to-night of the presentation of peace propositions from Gov [Joesph] Brown of Georgia to Sherman. Papers sell like hot cakes nowadays in the army. The soldiers hail with joy also the fall of gold "as it falls our wages rise" they all say. The Paymaster also is here and I shall soon send home some money, which I want invested in Uncle Sam bonds.

I did not intend to write much when I began and must close now and go to bed. I have hay for a bed and hay for a pillow, which is considered a luxury compared with Virginia feathers (alias pine boughs). My love to all as ever,

Your Affectionate Son
James D. Benton

PS Direct as usual

*   *   *   *

1st Div. Hospital
Oct 9, 1864

Dear Parents,

It is Sunday night and I am considerably lonesome so I thought I would write to you. I wrote to Maggie to-day and I might as well serve you the same while my hand is in.

---

19 Sherman's letter to Mayor James M. Calhoun, dated September 12, 1864, including the following line: "You cannot qualify war in harsher terms than I will. War is cruelty, and you cannot refine it; and those who brought war into our Country deserve all the curses and maledictions a people can pour out. I know I had no hand in making this war, and I know I will make more sacrifices to-day than any of you to Secure Peace." https://cwnc.omeka. chass.ncsu.edu/items/show/23, accessed September 19, 2017.

We are still in front of Petersburg and we have been here so long that I often wish we could get behind it as I think we will be in less than a month. I believe I gave you a description of my office and duties at the hospital in my last [letter] and repetition would be tiresome. We have moved the hospital lately and are now somewhat nearer the front. We are in plain sight of the city and country in its rear and can see the [rail] cars go out and come in from Richmond. We are just back of the high ground and by going forward a few rods we can see plainly all over the city, and the Rebel lines.

Our Regt. is now on the front line of works but we have had no men hurt very lately one or two wounded only come into the hospital daily. We are drawing the cords pretty close now around Petersburg and every stroke here is just as good as if it was executed directly on the Rebel capital. We have now a railroad all along the lines and it is only ten or twelve rods from where we are now located and it is the funniest railroad you ever saw. It goes up hill and down and all over it looks very queer to see a train go bobbing up and down the knolls as they do. The Johnnies have shelled it some but we throw up a protection for it and they have not tried it lately probably because they see it dont pay.

Petersburg is on low ground but after all it is not level ground but interspersed with hillocks and is quite a lengthy city lying along the Appomattox River. About ¾ or half a mile from it the ground gradually rises and then [in] back of that descends again and from the top of this elevation a plain view of all the surrounding country can be had, also of the city which however is a little obscured by a small piece of woods near our lines. It is surprising to see how much timber land there is here. We dont find any cities north containing 20,000 inhabitants as did Petersburg with timber land growing right up to within half a mile of it and all the region around covered with timber although not of the best quality. It is mostly pine but some oak hickory, cottonwood and sweet gum.

Did you ever think how singular it is that from the mouth of [the] James River to Richmond with the exception of City Point[20] (where there is two or three houses) that all along its banks of most delightful land and scenery

20 City Point was a river port at the junction of the James and Appomattox rivers. During the Civil War, it served as General Grant's headquarters throughout the Petersburg operations. In order to supply the Union army, two large military installations were erected there, one a supply depot and the other a field hospital. During the Petersburg operations, City Point was perhaps the busiest port in all of America.

there is not a village that could be called a corners. Compare it with the Hudson [River] and it is just as beautiful a river and you can see the legitimate results of the institution of human slavery.

But I am stringing out this letter to a considerable length and must close. I never was in better health in my life than now. I have expected a letter from you but it has not come as yet. I did not get paid as expected and as Uncle Sam is good and [the price of] gold falling, I am not afraid of national bankruptcy and the money will be just as good next payday as now. Lincoln will get the votes of the soldiers and that will do more to end the war than a great victory.

My love to all and I must bid you good night. Write soon and often I think Pa is a little dilatory about writing, it cant be pressure of business for I believe he did not take out a licence. Good Night.

Yours Affectionately
James D. Benton

P.S. Direct as usual.

*   *   *

October 18th 1864

Dear Parents,

It is considerable time since I last heard from you and I had contemplated writing before this and should have done so, only I was anticipating a letter from you consequently the delay.

I am still as when I last wrote in the Division hospital where I will probably remain sometime. I like my position very much. The siege of Petersburg still is in progress but no very active operations are transpiring just now except occasional shelling which was quite heavy last night. From our hospital we can see the mortar[21] shells sailing through the air in every

---

21 A mortar is a short, stout cannon designed to throw shells into fortifications by elevating the muzzle. The high elevation of the muzzle puts a large amount of strain on the gun, which is the reason the barrel is forged so short and thick. Because of the arc of the shell, mortars

direction sometimes a dozen at a time and the explosions make the earth shake.

The prospect is however that a movement will soon occur that will result in the capture of the two cities [Petersburg and Richmond] for which the contest has continued so long. I should not be surprised if this army cut loose from its base at City Point temporarily and by going around to the left secure the only remaining communication for the Rebels. If so, they must either starve in Richmond or come out and fight us, which they cannot do without entrenchments.

We are as an army in the most effective condition we ever were and it is astonishing what an immense number of recruits are coming to us. They have been arriving every day for the past month and at this time the trains go by almost every hour loaded with troops. Day after day they came pouring in.[22]

Everything looks like a move in a few days still it may be delayed some time though indications suggest the opposite opinion. Great enthusiasm exists not alone in regard to the election but as to military sucesses, which have of late been so [indecipherable]. Voting here is nearly over and there has not been as much noise about it in the whole army as will be in the Village of Ira on Election Day. But let the shelling commence and if we make some good shots they will cheer from one end of the line to the other regardless of political candidates. Lincoln will get a large majority of the army vote. Out of about 500 men there will be in our Regt. 50 McClellan votes. All will not do as well in this respect as our Regt. but if the election of Abraham depended on the soldier vote he might as well look up a boarding place in Washington for four years more. There is no doubt of his triumph. Copperheads are very scarce about here indeed.[23]

Beautiful weather, cool and pleasant, roads dusty, and as the boy said "a good ways from home" but we all live in hopes that the campaign of this

---

can drop a round into a fort or behind an entrenchment, whereas a cannon ball would either strike the outside or pass above it.

22 Tens of thousands of men were drafted or enlisted to replace the heavy losses suffered by the Union Army of the Potomac that summer and fall. The quality of these late-war arrivals was significantly less than their early-war counterparts, and veterans often looked down at the new arrivals.

23 Dr. Benton was correct—the army turned out in overwhelming support for President Lincoln, who nationwide garnered 2,218,388 votes overall to McClellan's 1,812,807. This translated into 212 electoral votes to 21.

fall will wind up the establishment of [Jefferson] Davis & Co. and that the books will be balanced. If there is any man in the world that I almost worship it is A. Lincoln and his executive conduct is unexceptionable. But I think he did make a little mistake when he wrote the letter headed, "To whom it may concern" inasmuch as making the abolition of Slavery a condition of returning allegiance. This war was undertaken as he proclaimed and as the people desired solely for the restoration of the Union and the reestablishment of its authority in the States, which had taken up arms against it. Now when that object is accomplished the purpose of this war is fulfilled and it ought to stop, and I think he makes a mistake when he adds the "abolition of slavery" as another condition and a condition he has no authority to make and which shuts the door of negotiations. He has no more power now to abolish slavery by proclamation in any southern state than he would have were there no war and when the war ceases the status of the State remains unchanged. No power except the State Legislature or Congress can abolish slavery. Military power will do it temporarily only. I think this the only blunder he has made. The expression did no good and precluded all hope of terms of peace. All we want in my opinion is that the Rebels lay down their arms and return to their allegiance to the Government and when they do that they have fulfilled all the conditions necessary and the object of this strife is entirely accomplished. Instead of the abolition of slavery the President might just as consistently with the Constitution and laws made the laying of an Atlantic telegraph by them one of the conditions of peace.

Slavery is dead if peace is declared in 24 hours but if it exists forever this war ought to stop when they lay down their arms and not until their [indecipherable] of that institution. I desire of course that its destruction as a war measure should ensure wherever the Union Army goes. Keep the slave from producing food to the advantage of the Rebellion, clean out the institution wherever we go but let the war end without any other conditions than the cessation of hostilities by them and the resumption of their fealty to the Government.

But I have splurged away considerably in this letter and it may be uninteresting and I will close it up. My love to all a wedding is close at hand I suppose over the way. Write often Pa has nothing else to do but write to me.

Your Affectionate Son
James D Benton

P.S. I have sent my vote to Heman and wish him to see it safely in the ballot box on the 8th of Nov. It contains a bullet for the Rebels and a ballot for Honest Old Abe. My love to all. J.D.B

*   *   *

111th N.Y.V.[24]
Nov. 6th 1864

Dear Parents,

Yours of the 28th was duly received and I do not know as I can conscientiously differ with you as far as political matters are concerned. I am sure at least that I sent a Lincoln vote to Heman to vote for me and that will speak for itself on the 8th.

You wanted to know something about the sick and wounded. We have not had many wounded lately but have in our hospital about 140 men sick and we receive probably three our four wounded per day for the reason that our Division is not now in the trenches but are now used as a support or reserve. They came out a day or two since and are having a chance to stretch themselves. A few Regts of the Division are still in the front line. The most prevalent diseases now are intermittent fever and diarrhea and we have comparatively few cases of serious illness.

We have one case which is worth relating to you. While the demonstration was being made on the Weldon Rail Road a short time since our Division held the line in front of Petersburg and the enemies line being much weakened we drove them out of one of their forts and occupied it an hour or two but were finally obliged to retreat from it. This man did not get back to our line as soon as the rest and the firing got to be so heavy that he had to lay down in a hole to save his life the lines only being a very short distance apart and skirmishing has been kept up ever since so much so that he staid in that hole eight days with no food except a few crumbs of hardtack he happened to have with him and no water but what fell from heaven. He did not dare to raise his head day or night from the hole for it would especially by

---

24 In November, the 111th New York was transferred to the 3rd Brigade, 1st Division, II Corps until the regiment was mustered out in June 1865.

day have been certain death. He lay until he could endure it no longer and as death was certain if he staid he took the only chance he had of running and came in all right. He is now in the hospital with gangrene of one of his feet as a consequence of his exposure. May the North only realize as far as possible that the constant watch of their faithful soldiers keep their lands and homes from devastation and ruin. It is precisely the same as if we were protecting you while you sleep and distance does not change the fact.

It is quite probable that the movement on the left was a reconnaissance in force and preparatory to a more earnest move, which will undoubtedly take place in a few days for it is quite evident that a great strike will soon come off. It is delayed in consequence of the Election in order that it might not have an unfavorable influence in case of a reverse. It is also generally opined that a change in the military commanders will soon take place. Hancock is going to leave our Corps where he will go is unknown. [25]

It may surprise you some if I tell you that the Commanding General of the Army of the Potomac and his staff subordinates are considerably Cooperish in their sentiments. I know it to be so from unquestionable authority and it is probably in consequence of jealousy instead of political difference. They are hostile to Hancock & the 2nd Corps and would do most anything to tarnish his or its good reputation. There will soon be a change and whatever it may be it will be welcome. Genl Meade's heart is not in this matter since Grant assumed his position. I think you may look for stirring news during the next two weeks.

But I must close. I hear that Jessie has been sick how is she? I trust she may soon recover. Before I write again I hope to hear a big sound from the ballot boxes of northern patriots. Write as soon as possible. I have much anxiety for Jessie but know she is in good hands.

As Ever
Your Affectionate Son
James D Benton

P.S. Tell Maggie to be sure and send me $1.00 worth of postage stamps.

---

25 General Hancock never fully recovered from a wound he received in the groin area at Gettysburg on July 3, 1863. By November 1864 he was exhausted, his wound was still painful and seeping, and he resigned from active service at the head of his II Corps.

1865

By the late fall of 1864, it was more than clear the Confederacy would lose the war. General Grant's aggressive style had kept General Lee's once feared Army of Northern Virginia locked into the trenches surrounding Richmond and Petersburg since June. Although his army was still powerful, Lee's command was shrinking with the passage of each day. In late June, Lee had detached Jubal Early's Corps to operate in the Shenandoah Valley, threaten Washington, and protect his own army's supply lines, for the Valley was his granary and without it his army would suffer greatly. Grant also dispatched reinforcements there and placed Phil Sheridan in command. A string of Southern defeats that fall in the Valley ended Confederate control of the Shenandoah.

General Sherman also maintained his relentless drive southward. Atlanta fell on September 1. After stripping Atlanta of what he needed, Sherman torched part of the city and set out toward Savannah on his March to the Sea. After capturing Savannah and offering it to President Lincoln as a Christmas president, two months later he set out northward into the Carolinas, where more hard fighting awaited. Sherman's former Confederate opponent, the Army of Tennessee, marched north into Tennessee under Gen. John Bell Hood and was sharply defeated at Franklin at the end of November and in the middle of December outside Nashville. What was left of his army retreated into Mississippi.

Throughout this period James Benton continued treating the wounded and sick of his 111th New York regiment from the area around Petersburg.

Only four letters during the last few months of the war have been located. He penned all four after his appointment to surgeon of the 98th New York Infantry Regiment.[1] He was commissioned surgeon on February 25, 1865, and served in that capacity from March 9 until August 31, 1865 when he was mustered out with the regiment at Richmond, Virginia.

*   *   *

Washington D.C.
March 5th 1865
Dear Parents,

It is Sunday and as I am considerably lonesome and a little homesick too. I guess I thought I would write a few lines at least to let you know how I am and where I am. As I am in anything but a writing mood you must excuse my brevity and poor writing. Now for my adventures.

I called on the Surgeon General of the Empire State and was politely informed by the Clerk of the Bureau that the state had favored me by issuing a commission making me a Surgeon of the 98th Regt. N.Y.V. I was a little surprised but easily recovered from it. Called at the Adjutant Generals Office and obtained my sheepskin. Now I am entirely satisfied and am willing to leave Uncle Sams employ most anytime. I shall try to not muster in for 3 years whether I can accomplish it or not I do not now know.

Well I arrived in this city in due time and reported to the Surgeon General U.S.A. who gave me permission to remain in town until the 7th still I

1   The 98th New York was raised in early 1862 with Colonel William Dutton, Lieutenant Colonel Charles Durkee and Major Albon Mann, as its field officers. It was made part of the 3rd Brigade, 3rd Division, 4th Army Corps, Army of the Potomac, and participated in the Peninsula Campaign and Seven Days' Battles outside Richmond that spring and summer. Colonel Dutton died of typhus that July and Lt. Col. Durkee was promoted to lead the regiment, which was transferred to Naglee's brigade in the Department of North Carolina. In early 1863 it was assigned to the 18th Army Corps and saw light action and garrison duty for most of the year. In 1864, the regiment moved with the corps northward and participated in Butler's Bermuda Hundred Campaign that May, and then in heavy actions north of the James River including Cold Harbor. The 98th participated in the Petersburg campaign and in December was transferred to the 1st Brigade, 3rd Division, 24th Army Corps. By the time the war ended, the regiment had lost two officers and 61 enlisted men killed in action, two officers and 37 enlisted men wounded, and four officers and 132 enlisted men died from disease. Frederick Phisterer, *New York in the War of the Rebellion, 1861-1865*, 6 vols. (J. B. Lyon Company, 1912), vol. 3, 3128.

think I shall go on to-morrow. I saw the Inauguration[2] and it was a very pretty sight but I could not get near enough to hear anything that was said without danger of suffocation by the crowd. An immense number of people were present from all parts of the U.S. and also from foreign countries. The descriptions of the ceremonies in the papers can explain it much better than I can so I refer you to them for the particulars. Abraham's address was very short but to the point. I am of the opinion that the occasion called for a more lengthy one. Still, I doubt not but what he understood his own business best.[3]

The morning was rather rainy and unpleasant enough, but the west was clear and just as Abraham made his appearance on the platform the sun burst into view and continued bright all day. This is one of the good omens.[4] Another is that during the afternoon a bright star made its appearance although the sun shone bright and the sky was clear, this is another [omen] and you can attach whatever importance to them you wish. I never saw a bright star in the daytime before.

Well I must stop as I must write to Maggie also to-day. You had better not write to me until I get located when I will give you directions. My love to all. Good Bye.

Your Affectionate Son
J. Dana Benton
Surgn 98th N.Y.V.

*   *   *

2   Dr. Benton is referring to the second inauguration of President Abraham Lincoln on March 4, 1865. The election of 1864 itself was rather remarkable given that the nation was in the midst of a long and bloody civil war. For the first and thus far only time, a portion of America did not officially participate in the election. Alabama, Arkansas, Florida, Georgia, Louisiana, Mississippi, North Carolina, South Carolina, Tennessee, Texas, and Virginia did not cast votes.

3   Like his Gettysburg Address, Lincoln's Second Inaugural Address was rather short, but it is also held out as perhaps his finest speech, and one of the best political speeches ever delivered.

4   Omen or not, it has been established that actor John Wilkes Booth attended the Second Inaugural Address. Lincoln was attending a play at Ford's Theatre in Washington on April 14, 1865, when he was shot in the back of the head by Booth and died the following morning in a boarding house across the street. He was the first American president to be assassinated.

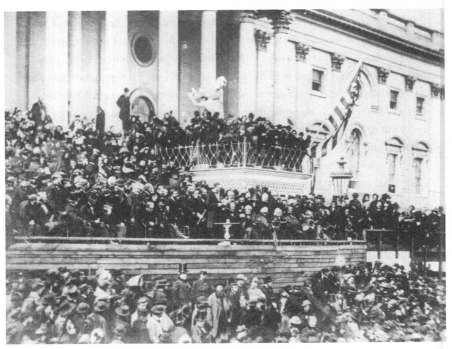

Abraham Lincoln delivering his second inaugural address on March 4, 1865. *LOC*

On April 1, 1865, a large mixed-arms strike force under Maj. Gen. Phil Sheridan was operating beyond the Union army's left flank and attacked an important intersection of roads called Five Forks. It was part of a larger effort to reach the Southside Railroad, General Lee's last railroad leading into Petersburg, and severe it. Maj. Gen. George Pickett (made famous by a charge at Gettysburg on July 3, 1863, that usually bears his name), was in command at Five Forks. Pickett was heavily outnumbered. The attack swept away his defenders and turned Lee's turned right flank. Holding Petersburg and Richmond was now no longer possible.

When he received the news, General Grant ordered an attack all along the lines early the following morning on April 2. The large-scale attack saw some of the hardest fighting of the war, but it also collapsed the defending lines.

The Confederate army and government officials evacuated the Southern capital and Petersburg on April 2, 1865. Lee's desperate plan was to withdraw his army westward and slip around Grant's left flank to join up somewhere in southern Virginia or North Carolina with Confederate forces under Gen. Joe Johnston.

*   *   *

Hd Qrs. 98th N.Y. Vols
Richmond Va.
April 7th 1865

Dear Parents,

For the first time since my arrival in this city I have now found a leisure moment to write to you and let you know of my welfare. The fact is somewhat surprising too as I have had comparatively nothing to do still [I am] very busy all the time. The only apology I can make is that there was so much to see and hear that I could not do anything else.

I have written once to Maggie since we occupied the city and I sent Pa this morning a copy of the Richmond Whig printed however on Confederate paper but with Union hands. It gives a detailed account of the evacuation by the Rebels and the occupation by our troops and it is much better told than I possibly could do.[5] Our Regt is now doing provost guard duty[6] in the city and our Lieut. Col[7] is an Apt. Prov. Marshal. I think we will stay here a long time at least I hope so. The Regiment is quartered in a large market building and our headquarters are in the St. Charles Hotel on Main Street, which is the principle business St. in the city.[8]

---

5 Retreating Southern soldiers had orders to burn bridges across the James River, the armory buildings, and various warehouses with supplies, but the fires spread out of control, and significant portions of the city burned down. Union troops helped extinguish the flames.

6 Provost Guard duty meant the New York soldiers were responsible for law and order within the city, and acted like military police.

7 William H. Rogers, Frederick Phisterer, *New York in the War of the Rebellion*, 6 vols. (J. B. Lyon Company, State Printers: Albany, NY, 1912), vol. 6, 3140-3141.

8 The four-story stucco St. Charles Hotel was built in 1846 and converted into Hospital Number Eight in the summer of 1861. It stood at the corner of 15th and Main Street. The hotel was not among the finest in town, and was considered "out of style" by most local Richmonders.

I was as you may easily suppose among the first that entered the place. My grey mane took me in on a good fast gallop. My heart was in my mouth and I have swallowed nothing but gratitude for sometime. I cant describe our entry very well all I can remember was flags flying the streets lined with people of all shades of color shouting, crying, and clapping their hands and thanking the Lord for a sight of the Old Flag which drives suffering and oppression from its presence. I saw the Star Spangled Banner erected on the Rebel Capitol amid such shouts as Richmond never heard before. Even the Confederates here are glad we have come for they see now a prospect of being relieved from starvation. The state of society was most horrible murder and plunder being the order of the day. Now all is quiet and every man can attend to his own business if he wishes to do so.

The first night after we came I was told that it was more quiet in the city than [had been] for many months. Our soldiers quell all disturbances immediately and at the point of the bayonet if necessary, and the citizens all commend them for their orderly and gentlemanly behavior. The people are very hospitable and friendly to us and try in every way to make our stay pleasant. Through the "mystic tie" as Bobby Burns sang I have made the acquaintance of many of the F.F.Vs where I know I would always be welcome.[9] We have brought order out of the chaos beginning by rescuing the city from the flames. The foundries and principle warehouses are entirely destroyed but the dwelling houses mostly all saved. Richmond is a pretty city for a southern one and much larger than I supposed.

I am in the best of health and get along finely with my Regt. the officers and men being apparently well pleased with me and my treatment of them. I have captured two or three nice articles, which I hope to get home sometime or other. Maggie always wanted me to capture something and I have done it.

Well I must close my letter for the present and I shall hope to hear from you very soon. Give my love to all and direct as usual.

Your Affectionate Son,
J. Dana Benton
Surg 98th N.Y.V.
1st Brig 3d Division 24th Army Corps
Army of the James

---

9 "F.F.Vs" mean first familes of Virginia.

*   *   *

With the loss of Five Forks and the general Union assault early on the morning of April 2, the Confederates began evacuating the Southern capital and Petersburg. Lee's plan was to withdraw his army westward and slip around Grant's left flank to join up somewhere in southern Virginia or North Carolina with Confederate forces under Gen. Joe Johnston.

The operation proved impossible. Lee's army was too hungry, too tired, and was not able to march fast enough and fight hard enough to accomplish his goals. General Grant accepted Lee's surrender on April 9, 1865, at Appomattox Courthouse. Although the war would continue for some time farther south and west, for all intents and purposes the war was over.

*   *   *

Richmond Va.
May 12, 1865

Dear Parents,

Doubtless you will think it strange that I have not written to you before but I have a valid excuse for it. My health has been so bad that it was impossible for me to write only upon great necessity.

For a long time I was unable to sit up and was in a hospital where I could not get anyone to write for me as they were all entire strangers and mostly Confederates. I am almost entirely recovered now and am with my Regiment, which is in the country on the south side of the [James] River. I came to it more for the fresh air than anything else and together with exercise on horseback it has done wonders. My disease was dysentery, which precluded almost to actual inflammation of the bowels and for some days it appeared as if my case would not result favorably but I am thankful that it was otherwise.

We are in a delightful camp in the woods and have nothing in the world to do only to keep our camp clean and eat & sleep. I might if I felt more like writing give you a lengthy description of our surroundings but as we will probably all be home soon it will be more interesting by word of mouth so I defer it. I receive letters very often from Maggie since she has been sick she cant do anything else and I could almost wish she might linger along a little so I could hear so much oftener from home. I received last night a letter from

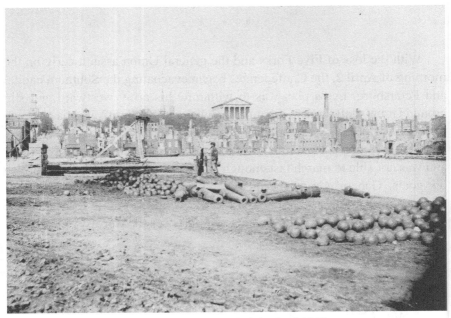

The ruins of Richmond, Virginia, April 1865. *NA*

Pa dated March 30th but there was not much news in it, still I think it prompted me to write to-day.

Well the war is over and I suppose you are all rejoicing over it. I know we are though there is an evident uneasiness among the soldiers to know what they will do when they get home and many are canvassing the prospects of gold in Mexico and many for a farm in Canada. The Mexican Government for pay can get enough men in three months to start the frog-eating Johnny Crapeau on a double quick for 'la belle France.''[10]

I am sorry to learn by Maggie's letter that Ma does not recover her usual strength and health. I wish you would give me particulars as to her

---

10 The word "crapaud" is a derogatory term for the French, who together with two other foreign countries, was a foreign creditor of Mexico. After President Benito Juárez suspended interest payments in mid-1861, Emperor Napoleon III of France invaded later that same year. He justified the act by arguing he was all in favor of free trade, and an allied government in Mexico would help France secure access to Central and South American markets. Mexico was also rich with silver, which Napoleon would need to fund his desires for overseas expansion. Napoleon built a coalition with Spain and Britain while the U.S. was deeply engaged in its civil war, which made it much easier fo them to do so.

case. I must stop now for dinner and I shall soon expect to hear from you. If Pa would send me some two-cent stamps I will send him the Richmond papers occasionally. Write soon.

Your Affectionate Son,
J. Dana Benton
Surg 98th NYV

*   *   *

Head Quarters 98th N.Y.V.
June 9th 1865

Dear Parents,

I received Pa's letter of the 4th last night and was considerably surprised to learn that you had not heard from me. It has been only a short time since I wrote to you but I presume that the letter has been lost or missent. I write immediately therefore to allay any apprehension that may be entertained as to my welfare.

I am in excellent health and were the weather not so excessively hot should be perfectly happy. It is uncommonly warm here for the season of the year. We still remain in the same place near Manchester, which is across the river from Richmond and in a pleasant though rather an unhealthy locality.

The mustering officers are busy mustering out all men whose time expires previous to Oct 1st next. This is constantly reducing our numbers and when it is completed we are to be consolidated so as to form two Brigades in the Division instead of three as they now exist. I do not know positively what Regiments will be united to us but we think the 139th N.Y. and the 118th [N.Y.][11] *and if so I will be retained as I rank their medical officers and it is*

---

11 On July 7, 1862, Colonel Samuel T. Richards received authority to recruit the 118th New York in the counties of Clinton, Essex, and Warren. It was organized at Plattsburg, New York and mustered in August 18-20, 1862. Members not discharged with the regiment were transferred to the 96th New York regiment on June 13, 1865. The regiment was mustered out under Colonel George F. Nichols on June 13, 1865 at Richmond, Virginia. During its service the regiment lost six officers and 286 enlisted men. https://dmna.ny.gov/historic/reghist/civil/infantry/118thInf/118thInfMain.htm.

favorable that after the super [indecipherable word] officers are mustered out I will be elevated to Brigade Surgeon an honorary, though no more profitable, position. I am more and more convinced that we will be retained for a considerable time yet and that impression appears to prevail among the greater mass of officers.

I am not sorry if it is so for I had as leave spend the summer in the army as not. I know I could not do as well in any business in the north. My pay now amounts to about $200 per month and if I remain until the Regiment goes out I will be entitled to three months extra pay. My months pay proper is $80 so I will get $240 extra.

Now Pa I wish you would do something for me. I am out of money and I want $100 sent to me by express. I dont know how long it will be before we are paid but there is no immediate prospect of it. I have plenty of money if it is so. It can be got as Maggie has notes; Charley Lees $500 and Maggie has some 7.30 bonds. I dont want to disturb that on which Charley has got if it can be helped. I prefer to have either a note collected or if you have the money you may take one of the 7.30 bonds and send me the money for it. I wish you would see Maggie and make arrangements to send it immediately as I am greatly in want of it. Have it sent by express directed as usual. They have envelopes at the express office for that purpose.

I wish Maggie would come down here and if you would come with her I would still be better pleased. But I must stop now and hope to hear from you soon.

My love to all

As Ever Yours
J. Dana Benton
Surg 98 N.Y.V.

*   *   *

James Benton was honorably discharged and mustered out of service on August 31, 1865 at Richmond, Virginia.

*   *   *

Alba Bradford Co. Pa
November 29, 1865

Dear Father,

Here I am in the midst of oildom and begin to feel greasy already.[12]
I reached here this (Thursday) morning and I am afraid S. E. Shepard will think I have commenced boring immediately for if I have not bored I certainly have pumped him with questions. I have also seen oil genuine, fresh oil right from the well all the question that can arise is as to the quantity that the well is going to afford. They struck it at a depth of 416 feet while the average depth of oil wells is about 600 feet. As soon as it was found they stopped and they have sent for tubing, which will be here in a few days and then they will commence pumping. There was a considerable sediment in the well at the time they stopped held in suspension by the meter and this has settled to the bottom which obstructs the oil. This will be bored out again previous to tubing. They obtained 3 or 4 pints of oil of about the consistence of good thick syrup and it is to be seen now on the pump and also on the water drawn from the well. I have not invested any yet but shall and I think there can be no failure for they will certainly sink at least two more wells whether this proves a success or not and that will keep the price of stock up.

The Dr. will not hear to my leaving at present and I may stay some little time. He is making my visit a very pleasant and instructive one. The well is about ¾ of a mile from the village (south) near a small stream, which runs through a gully between two rises of ground. The excitement has raised the price of village property about one half and land has raised from 40 & 50 to 100 dollars per acre in the vicinity. Of course oil is the only thing talked about through this section, still everyone seems to take the matter very cool and all seem to have great confidence in it those who have no immediate interest in it as well as those who have. The material facts are of course as the Dr. stated in his letters to you.

---

12 Unfortunately, there is no information about when James decided to travel to Pennsylvania or how he got there. The Benton family is unaware of any facts related to James's time sent prospecting for oil in the Keystone State.

Well I must close for the present if I stay long I will write again still I think I shall be home in a few days. Tell Maggie not to buy any more calico dresses and to be careful who she associates with. Good Bye.

Yours Affectionately

James D. Benton
Late of U.S.A now in the act of striking oil

* * *

Prior to the Civil War in the 1850s, the groundwork was being set for an industry that would revolutionize the world. The first process for refining crude oil was patented in England in 1850, and just a few years later a sample of petroleum from Titusville, Pennsylvania, was discovered and the Pennsylvania Rock Oil Company organized. There was money to be made in oil, especially when the beneficial properties and uses of petroleum were discovered.

A boom and bust cycle plagued the state's nascent oil industry until John D. Rockefeller organized Standard Oil and imposed order on the industry just a handful of years after James's dabbling in the industry. The invention of the light bulb and the widespread use of electricity replaced kerosene and threatened the oil industry, but the invention and popularity of the automobile increased the need for gasoline. Pennsylvania oil would come to dominate the market, directing the way to America's eventual reliance on petroleum.[13]

13 American Chemical Society National Historic Chemical Landmarks. Development of the Pennsylvania Oil Industry. www.acs.org/content/acs/en/education/whatischemistry/landmarks/pennsylvaniaoilindustry.html (accessed 09/25/2017).

Postscript

1885

With the surrender of General Lee's Army of Northern Virginia at Appomattox Court House on April 9, 1865, the Civil War in Virginia had reached its end. Johnston's Confederate army would surrender in North Carolina later that month to General Sherman, and other Rebel forces at various places across the South during the next month or so. Two months after Lee's capitulation, James and the remaining men of the 98th New York were transferred to the 2nd Brigade, 3rd Division, XXIV Corps in June, where they would remain until the end of their service. On August 31, 1865, James and comrades were honorably discharged and mustered out of service at Richmond, Virginia under Colonel William Kreutzer.

The remaining years of James's life are not as well known or documented. According to the New York State Census of 1865, he returned home to Ira, New York, where he was reunited with his wife Margaret and their daughter Jessie. As indicated by the previous letter dated November 29, 1865, he traveled to Pennsylvania, presumably lured by the excitement of the oil boom. Exactly what he was doing there, who he was with, or how long he remained is anyone's guess, for this is the only known correspondence from Pennsylvania; nothing else has surfaced in family records.

After his oil venture in the Keystone state, James once more returned home to Ira, presumably by the end of 1865. According to the *History of Cayuga County*, James had a medical practice in the town of Ira, New York,

JAS. D. BENTON, M. D.,

PHYSICIAN AND SURGEON,

OFFICE AND RESIDENCE,

Corner of Elbridge and Barrett Streets,

Fifth Ward,   **SYRACUSE, N. Y.**

Having had twenty years experience in Hospital, Army, and Private practice, I am prepared to attend any
cases entrusted to my care.
N. B.—DISEASES OF FEMALES MADE A SPECIALTY.

Office

Room No 1 Myers Block

A business card from his practice still exists. *Benton Family*

from 1865 until 1874, when he removed to Syracuse, New York and
continued his medical practice.[14] The New York State Census taken June 1,
1875, lists James, his wife Margaret, and their daughter Jessie living in
Syracuse. A United States Federal Census dated June 6, 1880, has James still
residing in Syracuse with his occupation as doctor.

*   *   *

By the 1880s, with the war and a significant portion of his life
behind him, James decided to address something that had been
eating at his conscience.

In early April 1865, he entered Richmond with other Union troops and
took up quarters at the St. Charles Hotel. There, he came across an
abandoned box of books with a Bible inside. James took it with him, and
kept it for twenty years. It was time to try and locate its original and rightful
owner and return it. He knew his name, and that the previous owner had been

---

14 Elliot G. Storke, *History of Cayuga County, With Illustrations and Biographical
Sketches of Some of its Prominent Men and Pioneers* (Syracuse, N.Y.: D. Mason, 1879),
296.

from Augusta, Georgia, so he wrote a letter to the postmaster of that city in the hope he could forward it on.

*　*　*

Cato NY.
June 13, 1885

P.M. Augusta Ga.

Dear Sir,

I am anxious to find persons by the name of Edgar Redden Derry, Rev[rend] W. J. Hard, or their nearest kin.

I have in my possession a family Bible that I preserved at the evacuation of Richmond from the depredation of those who would have destroyed it. I desire to restore it to its rightful owner if they desire it. It contains a family record, also an envelope containing the wedding cards of Edgar R. Derry and Julia A. Hard, and in the envelope is also a lock of hair evidently that of a child.

If you know of any such persons, please manage to put me in correspondence with them if you can and oblige.

Yours Respectfully,

James D. Benton M.D.
Cato, Cayuga Co. N.Y.

P.S. I was late surgeon of the 98th N.Y. Volunteers

*　*　*

To James's surprise, he received a speedy reply dated just ten days after he penned and mailed his original query. Undoubtedly he was also pleased by the deep level of detail contained in the letter.

*　*　*

Office Derry and Law
845 Broad St.
Augusta Ga.

June 23, 1885

Dr. James D. Benton
Cato, N.Y.

Dear Sir,

Your letter of inquiry of 19inst addressed to the P.M. [Postmaster] at this place was placed in our box by him, and so promptly reached my hand.

Permit me to thank you for your exceeding kindness, both in preserving what is to me a most sacred relic and in your endeavor to find its owner. This Bible was given to Julia A. Hard and myself by our cousin Prof[essor] J. T. Derry as a wedding present, he being my first groomsman. We were married as the card indicates the night after Mr. Lincoln was first elected President in 1860 (Nov.).

I was in Richmond the winter of 1864-5. I had a room at the St. Charles Hotel and in Feb 1865 lost my wife while there. She having fled from this place (Augusta Ga.) fearing that this city would fall into the hand of Gen. Sherman on his march to the sea—and had packed in a large box and trunk her clothing (and childs) with such valuables as she most valued and among which was this Bible.

When Richmond was evacuated on Sunday night Apr 2/65, I locked my room and left Richmond on the train, which brought out the [President Jefferson Davis] administration. In October following I returned to Richmond, went to the hotel, and the only information I could get concerning my effects was that Federal soldiers had opened and carried off the contents of the trunk and box.

If you can send me that precious book, which is beyond all value, I shall feel under lasting obligations to you and will gladly reward you for any expense you may have been subjected to. I can not begin to thank or express the thanks which I feel for I never more expected to hear of its whereabouts.

As I have already stated, my wife died in Feb. prior to the evacuation of Richmond in Apr. 1865, leaving to my care an infant of about seven months—that child (a girl) was married last Wednesday evening the 17inst.

If you will send me the Bible and the little relic by express and state the expense, I will remit check on N. York for it. I would be most glad if you would write me the history of your possession and care of the book for I know but little of what took place after I left the fallen city, or Capitol.

If you ever visit our sunny clime, and pass through this beautiful city I would be delighted to have you call on me. May I not hear from you soon?

Respectfully etc.

E. R. Derry

*   *   *

The original owner of the pilfered Bible, Edgar R. Derry, worked for Derry and Law, a grocery store in Augusta, Georgia. Edgar was born on January 1, 1835 in New Jersey, but was living in Augusta, Georgia, by 1854. How he came to reside in the deep South is anyone's guess.

There was no doubt where his sentiments rested, for he enlisted on April 10, 1862, in Augusta and served with the 12th Battalion, Georgia Light Artillery (also known as the Savannah Siege Train Heavy Artillery Battalion). That June, the command was assigned to the Department of South Carolina, Georgia, and Florida, and saw service at Fort McAllister in Savannah, Georgia, and Fort Sumter and Battery Wagner at Charleston, South Carolina. In May 1863, Edgar was transferred to Richmond, where he entered the hospital service to look after the sick and the wounded. He was discharged from service in February 1865 because of tuberculosis.[15]

James promptly penned a reply of his own.

*   *   *

15 The 12th Battalion, Georgia Light Artillery was transferred to the Army of Northern Virginia in May 1864, where it became part of General Clement A. Evans' Brigade. The artillerists served as infantry at Cold Harbor before transferring to the Shenandoah Valley to fight with Jubal Early's Valley army. The command returned and was present for the fall of Richmond and retreated to Appomattox, where six officers and 125 men surrendered. USGenWeb Archives, 12th Battalion Georgia Light Artillery, http://files.usgwarchives. net/ga/military/civilwar/rosters/12thbatt.txt.

Cato, N.Y.
June 26, 1885

E. R. Derry

Dear Sir,

Your letter of the 23rd in this morning received and I hasten to reply.

As far as I can I will give you the history of this Bible's wanderings. I was Surgeon of the 98th New York Volunteers, and at the evacuation [of Richmond] my regiment was camped at Chapin's [Chaffin's] farm just below the city. We went into Richmond on the morning of April 3rd or 4th and remained there about three weeks doing provost duty. While there our regimental headquarters were in the St. Charles Hotel and I occupied a room that contained a box of books (the trunk I never saw). Previous to my having the room it had been rummaged by soldiers, and this Bible was at the bottom of a box with small books on top, hence not discovered. In the confusion of our entrance it would have been carried away by soldiers who would have had no regard for its ownership, or entirely destroyed.

We went from Richmond to Burkesville, thence to Farmville, Va. where we remained three or four weeks, or until about the middle of August 1865, when we were ordered back to Richmond and on August 31st 1865 were mustered out. This Bible accompanied me and to my wife who joined me at Richmond soon after our entry and who was with me all that summer is due the credit of its preservation. I was taken violently sick while in the St. Charles Hotel, and was cared for by a Confederate Surgeon, a Dr. Aiken or Aken of Georgia.

We were sent to New York after our discharge and after coming home the Bible and its owner were a frequent topic of conversation, which generally ended in the conclusion that those concerned were probably dead or never to be found. I kept it seven years at my home in Cato, then ten years in Syracuse, N.Y. and last spring brought it with me to Cato, where it now is, and it shall be properly boxed and sent to you immediately.

I am only too sorry that two or three entries in the record of my own family have been made, but I thought it better not to erase or mutilate it and let you do as you prefer. In the record you will find the wedding card and the lock of hair, which I know you will prize highly. The book is in a fair state of preservation. The stains are from water while kept in a tent, and the natural wear it would incur during twenty years.

My dear sir, I am only too glad to return the book to its rightful owner. The war and three years of service have made me a physical wreck, and although I get a small pension from the Government, it can never restore health and strength and it only remains for me to do an act of justice. In the hope that the blue and gray may every passing year be connected closer in the bonds of friendship, which should unite brave men to defend and perpetuate a Republic that will be forever an ornament and blessing to the world and civilization, I remain, very respectfully yours—

James D. Benton

*   *   *

With the Bible now safely back in the rightful owner's hands, James's conscience was clean and the matter ended there. Edgar's life, however, had several twists and turns, including an unfortunate event during his final few years.

The aging Derry, whom an Augusta newspaper described as "one of the most highly respected and esteemed men of Augusta, Georgia," became the treasurer and secretary of the Augusta Real Estate and Building Association. When an audit was performed in 1906, the records were found in shambles and thousands of dollars unaccounted for. It was clear the former soldier was not up to the task of running the operation and had not personally benefitted, but a grand jury had no choice but to indict him for embezzlement. Derry himself was broke and "brooded over the matter in sorrow." Even those who had lost money because of his negligence did not think he had intentionally stolen it, and no one wanted to press the case.

And there the matter lingered for several years. It might have faded away altogether except for Derry himself, who appeared before the judge at the age of 79 against the advice of friends and relatives to explain that the mattered "weighed" on him and that "he must pay in some way to those who had lost before death claimed him." A reluctant judge accepted his guilty plea and sentenced him to a year in jail under circumstances that can only be described as both heartbreaking and extraordinary. He served his time and was released. The same judge who had sentenced him sought a pardon, and the governor of Georgia signed it "to remove any stain from his name and restore him to full citizenship."

According to his son, W. R. Derry, the elderly Derry died suddenly and unexpectedly on March 7, 1923.[16]

*   *   *

It is unknown when James moved his practice from Syracuse back to Cato. According to an update on the Albany Medical school class of 1857, James was practicing medicine in Cato, New York in 1887, though no records thereafter have surfaced.[17]

James was still living in Ira and practicing medicine according to the New York State Census taken February 16, 1892. A few months later, on May 16, 1892 at the age of 54, he passed away. He is buried in Union Hill Cemetery, Cato, NY.

16 Undated newspaper clipping entitled "Governor Pardons Edgar R. Derry on Plea of Citizens."

17 J. Montgomery Mosher, M.D., ed., *Albany Medical Annals, Journal of the Alumni Association of the Albany Medical College*, Vol XXVIII (Press of Brandow Printing Co: Albany, NY, 1907), 539. Almost all of the United States Federal Census of 1890 was destroyed by a fire at the Commerce Department in Washington, D.C. on January 10, 1921. Surviving fragments consists of 1,233 pages or pieces, and the records of only 6,160 of the 62,979,766 people covered by the census survive. The records for James and his family are not among them.

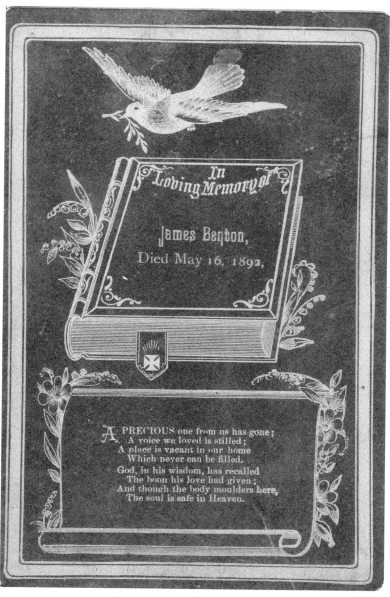

James's memorial card. *Benton Family*

Appendix A

Dr. Jonathan Letterman: Architect of Battlefield Triage

Although Camp Fitzgerald was nothing like pretty little Fort Tejon in the Tehachapi Mountains north of Los Angeles, it was where Captain and Assistant Surgeon Jonathan Letterman was ordered to go. He accompanied the dragoons in his care down to the new campsite, but no one was prepared for the dust, dirt, and the lack of water and pasture for horses.[1] South Carolina's Fort Sumter had been attacked six weeks ago, and times were uncertain. Dr. Letterman must have longed for the opportunity to go where he could do more than simply serve in far western postings where mobile medical units accompanied small units of soldiers in their attempts to control the Indians.

In his introduction to *Death, Disease, and Life at War*, author-editor Chris Loperfido mentions the desertion to the Confederacy of three Federal army surgeons and twenty-one assistant surgeons. Doctor Jonathan Letterman was not one of them. By December 1861, Letterman had been ordered to New York City. After ten years in the West, he was now a medical purveyor in charge of purchasing supplies for the army medical department, which had been inundated by orders for the surge of manpower announced by President Lincoln. However, Letterman had just gotten his forms in order when another transfer came through. January 1862 found the tall, thin Letterman installed as Medical Director in the Department of West Virginia. He was paired up with Dr. William Hammond, the highly intelligent,

---

1 www.militarymuseum.org/CpFitzLA.html (accessed April 3, 2017).

oversized personality who would soon become the Union's Surgeon General shortly before Letterman took over as Medical Director of the Army of the Potomac. Both men were finally in positions to make progress in the field of medicine that was simply astonishing in its depth, complexity, and value.[2]

Federal military forces grew from about 16,000 soldiers in 1859 to hundreds of thousands in answer to President Lincoln's call for more men on July 22, 1861.[3] The need for a functional medical system to care for these fighting forces was imperative. Until July 1862, this effort was marred by outdated methods and ideas, personal animosities, and a lack of vision. Jonathan Letterman's creation of a fully operational system of battlefield evacuation and care for the Army of the Potomac, based on logistics and focused on the needs of the soldiers in the field, all in eighteen months, was nothing less than amazing.

Considering the damage done by the firepower of an army through casualties, most generals were anxious to see a system promoting health and adequate care of the wounded. Logistics played the most important role in battlefield evacuation. The medical evacuation system Letterman designed—battlefield triage—started right on the battlefield with an immediate analysis of the severity of injury. This led to progressive stations of care designed to move the most critical cases along the fastest, organized a hospital staff to best deal with the wounded, designed a transportation system to send the wounded to the most appropriate care, and demanded that surgeons keep records to forward with the patient to accelerate their care. To think that these rudimentary methods were absent in American armies before 1862 is appalling, but it was true.

Hammond, now Surgeon General, appointed Letterman to be Medical Director of the Army of the Potomac in July 1862. The doctor arrived at Harrison's Landing and found within a week of his arrival the generally deplorable conditions confronting the Army Medical Department. Letterman's immediate concern was the health of the men who were not wounded, but ill. Letterman compared the geography surrounding

---

2 Scott McGaugh, *Surgeon in Blue: Jonathan Letterman, the Civil War Doctor Who Pioneered Battlefield Care* (New York: Arcade Publishing, 2013), 48-74.

3 US Army Center of Military History, "The Civil War-1861," American Military History, v.1, ch. 9, www.history.army.mil/books/AMH-V1/ch09.htm, 213 (accessed June 14, 2017).

Harrison's Landing to a "Serbonian Bog," and proceeded to make inroads into rescuing the health of McClellan's army. He wrote:

> This marching and fighting in such a region, in such weather, with lack of food, want of rest, great excitement, and the depression necessarily consequent upon it, could have no other effect than that of greatly increasing the numbers of sick after the army reached Harrison's Landing.[4]

After estimating that the number of sick amounted to over 20% of the army, he put down his pencil and went to work. Jonathan Letterman, now Major Letterman, asked Hammond for 1,000 hospital tents and 200 ambulances to move and shelter the thousands of sick and wounded soldiers who had not been given anything resembling medical care since being brought in from the battlefields near Richmond during the Seven Days' Battles (June 25-July 1, 1862). Hammond quickly sent the required tents and ambulances. Letterman commandeered several buildings, including the beautiful Berkeley plantation, to be used as hospitals and places of respite until the tents arrived.

On July 2, Surgeon General Hammond's hospital ships began to show up. They were fitted with beds, bedding, medicines, hospital supplies, food—everything that was needed for the comfort and well being of the wounded and seriously ill. The loading and shipment of these men started immediately, and continued until the docks at Harrison's Landing had been cleared. By July 15, more than 7,000 soldiers had been sent to hospitals at Fortress Monroe and other places North. This could not have been accomplished without the joint cooperation of Surgeon General Hammond and the U.S. Sanitary Commission volunteers, with whom a strong bond had been forged.[5] Dr. James D. Benton notes this bond in his letter of June 5, 1864.

After little more than a month as Medical Director, Letterman prepared and McClellan approved the Army of the Potomac's Special Order No. 147 of August 2, 1862. This order laid the foundations for the organization and operation of ambulances in the Union Army. Letterman had already

---

4 Jonathan Letterman, *Medical Recollections of the Army of the Potomac* (Bedford, Massachusetts: Applewood Books reprint, 1866), 7.

5 Ibid., 8-9, 10-11.

witnessed first hand the disorganization and rampant misuse of the field ambulances under the purview of the Quartermaster Corps. The typical Civil War ambulance of 1861-62 was a two-wheeled cart with no springs, known derisively as the "Avalanche." They were too few, too far between, and mostly too late. Ambulance drivers were almost always civilians, sometimes drunk, sometimes thieves, and often cowards who left their coach seats when the guns began to fire. Many men were jarred to death by the ride in an ambulance. The North abandoned this type of transportation within the first year of the war, as most of the 2-wheelers had broken down beyond repair within a few months of service.[6] The 4-wheel Rucker model ambulance, a much softer ride for the wounded, replaced the old "Avalanche."[7]

The sixteen provisions of Special Orders No. 147 detailed the organization of the ambulance corps and the management of ambulance trains. It assigned officers to the Ambulance Corps who were not part of the Quartermaster Corps. Drivers were chosen from the ranks, and were to be drilled in their unique duties. Teams of horses or mules were designated as belonging to the Ambulance Corps, and were not to be requisitioned by anyone else for any other purposes. Tack and feed were the properties of the Ambulance Corps, as were all the accouterments necessary inside the ambulances and transport carts. The responsibilities for keeping the gear in perfect order was spelled out. Most importantly, these orders allowed the Ambulance Corps to function as its own entity, no longer dependent on the Quartermaster Corps for anything. "The Captain is the commander of all the ambulances and transport carts in the Army Corps, under the direction of the Medical Director."[8] This gave the surgeons and other medical staff the support necessary to do their job. Their insignia consisted of—for privates, a green band, 2 inches broad, around the cap, a green half-chevron, 2 inches broad, on each arm above the elbow. Non-commissioned officers wore the same band around the cap, and full chevrons.[9] With the issuance of a single

6 Katherine Traver Barkley, *The Ambulance: The Story of Emergency Transportation of Sick and Wounded Through the Centuries* (Kiamesha Lake, New York: Load N Go Press, 1990), 25.

7 Ibid., 27.

8 Letterman, *Medical Recollections of the Army of the Potomac*, 24-30.

9 Ibid.

order, Jonathan Letterman redefined battlefield evacuation from a post-battle scavenger hunt to one marked by military discipline and order.[10]

McClellan would later write of Letterman: "I saw immediately that Letterman was the man for the occasion, and at once gave him my unbounded confidence . . . I never met with his superior in power of organization and executive ability."[11]

At Antietam, Letterman's plan for battlefield triage—the orderly and efficient system for the treatment and evacuation of wounded soldiers—was used for the first time. It began right on the firing lines, where regimental surgeons were the first responders. Men thought to have mortal wounds were made as comfortable as possible and left to die or evacuated last. Wounded men were brought from the battlefield on stretchers along Letterman's pre-determined routes to often-crude field hospitals. At each field hospital, "dressers" performed basic triage, sorting men for treatment by the severity of their wounds. After being stabilized, most patients were transported by ambulance to division hospitals located toward the rear of the battlefield. Letterman created two long-term tent hospitals at Antietam – the first of their kind – at Smoketown and Keedysville.[12] Soldiers were given intensive care at this point. Wounds were carefully cleaned and explored, bones were set, and amputations were performed. After a period of brief rest, both the seriously and not so seriously wounded were moved by ambulance, train, or hospital ship to long-term recovery hospitals in Frederick, MD and Washington. The hospitals created for the Battle of Antietam were largely empty by October.[13] Before Antietam, before Jonathan Letterman, no medical evacuation plan of any type had ever been considered. Today, Letterman's plan remains fundamental in handling battlefield casualties and critical national and international emergencies.

Not everything worked perfectly in this inaugural outing of Letterman's triage plans. There was miscommunication and mistakes were made. Lack of supplies was the greatest problem the Medical Corps faced at Antietam. The

---

10 *OR* 23, pt. 1, 217.

11 John T. Greenwood, "Hammond and Letterman: A Tale of Two Men Who Changed Army Medicine," *An Institute of Land Warfare Publication* (San Antonio, Texas, June 2003), 3.

12 www.civilwarmed.org/letterman-dinner/letterman-father-of-battlefield-medicine/.

13 Letterman, *Medical Recollections of the Army of the Potomac*, 50-51.

Army of the Potomac's supply system became jammed at Frederick and Baltimore and desperately needed medical supplies failed to reach the battlefield until days after the fighting. Unfortunately, some care sites had been erected on the field unbeknownst to Letterman or his staff. These went unattended for lengthy periods of time. Besides the supply issues, Jonathan Letterman's authority did not extend to refusing to let families take wounded sons, brothers, or fathers out of the field hospitals he had worked so hard to establish. He knew his patients were probably going to a less healthy environment. He knew the chances were good that the soldier would not even survive the trip home. He could do nothing about McClellan's orders that some state relief societies could take their men home as well. Because of these removals, thousands of soldiers were lost to the Army of the Potomac. Their return to duty was uncertain, at best.[14]

The sanitation hazards of the dead and dismembered could not be ignored. Nearly a week after the Battle of Antietam, the dead were still not buried. The charnel stench was much written about. "I have seen, stretched along in one line, ready for interment, at least 1,000 blackened, bloated corpses with blood and gas protruding from every orifice and maggots holding high carnival over their heads," wrote the 121st New York's assistant surgeon Daniel M. Holt.[15] It is little wonder that Dr. Benton did not write home to his parents or wife concerning the terrible sights he saw on a daily basis.

Nevertheless, after Antietam, Letterman continued to develop a field hospital system that would properly care for the sick and wounded. In October 1862 he revamped the organization for ordering and delivering medical supplies. He also fleshed out the field hospital structure. Both systems would be continually refined throughout the war. In four short months, from July through October 1862, Letterman set the foundation for the complete rebuilding of the organization and administration of the Union Army's field medical system. Later he wrote:

> It will be perceived that the ambulance system, with that of supplies and of field hospitals, were ordered as essential parts of that new organization

---

14 McGaugh, *Surgeon in Blue*, 120.

15 James M. Greiner, ed., *A Surgeon's Civil War: The Letters and Diary of Daniel M. Holt, M. D.* (Ohio: Kent State University Press, 1994). 38.

from which, I earnestly hoped, the wounded and sick would receive more careful attendance and more skillful treatment.[16]

Following the battles of Chancellorsville and Gettysburg, Letterman codified the changes he had made in battlefield emergency care in the Army of the Potomac's General Order No. 85, issued August 24, 1863. Congress finally took this General Order and modified it into the act of March 11, 1864. This act established Letterman's system throughout the Union Army and forever changed the Army Medical Department.[17]

Although Major Jonathan Letterman left the Union army on December 22 1864, during his tenure as medical director for the Army of the Potomac he was able to bring about tremendous change from practices of the past. Letterman's legacy continues to inspire medical military personnel as his innovations in military and emergency medical care made during the American Civil War continue today, from homeland emergency preparedness, to the care and treatment of service members serving in such dangerous places as the Middle East.

Major General Paul R. Hawley, chief surgeon, European Theater of Operations, said, "There was not a day during WWII that I did not thank God for Jonathan Letterman. He was truly a surgeon for the soldiers."[18] That a general officer in WWII should still be impressed with a Civil War doctor strikes one as deceptively important. This feeling continues today, as Dr. Jonathan Letterman's basic plan for battlefield triage has had no problem evolving into the 21st century. Perhaps horses no longer pull the ambulances, but the medics on the helicopters are carrying Letterman's work forward.

by Meg Groeling

author of *The Aftermath of Battle:*
The Burial of the Civil War Dead (Savas Beatie, 2015)

---

16 Letterman, *Medical Recollections of the Army of the Potomac*, 63-64.

17 General Orders No. 106 War Department, Adj. General's Office "Uniform System of Ambulances" (Washington, March 16, 1964). See http://civilwarhome.com/congress ambulanceact.htm.

18 Kyle Wichtendahl. "Dr. Jonathan Letterman: Father of Modern Medicine," www.civil warmed.org/letterman-dinner/letterman-father-of-battlefield-medicine/.

Appendix B

The U.S. Sanitary Commission During the Civil War

"These cookies are expressly for the sick soldiers, and if anyone else eats them, I hope they will choke him"

On Friday, March 18, 1864, the Washington D.C. Sanitary Fair was closing. The event was graced by the appearance of President Lincoln who, in his closing remarks, mentioned, "If all that has been said by orators and poets since the creation of the world in praise of women applied to the women of America, it would not do them justice for their conduct during this war."[19] To much applause, Lincoln finally gave attention to the original founders of the United States Sanitary Commission.

Originally created as the Women's Central Association of Relief (WCAR), it began in New York City under the guiding hands of Dr. Elizabeth Blackwell. Blackwell wanted to "organize the whole benevolence of women in the country into a general and central association," according to USSC nurse and historian Katherine Wormeley. The WCAR would coordinate and organize the local relief efforts of all northern women, communicate directly with the Army's medical department about the soldiers' needs, and perform the selection, registration, and training of women nurses.[20] But the WCAR ran into trouble almost immediately. Army

19 "Remarks at Closing of Sanitation Fair," (Washington, D.C., March 18, 1864), in Roy P. Basler, ed., *The Collected Works of Abraham Lincoln*, 8 vols. (Rutgers U. Press, 1953), vol. 3, 254.

20 Katherine Wormeley, *The United States Sanitary Commission: A Sketch of its Purposes and Work* (Boston: Little, Brown and Company, 1863), 3.

medical officer Dr. R.C. Satterlee believed that the group, composed of elite Northern women used to having their demands met, would be "obtrusive."[21] Satterlee merely mirrored the opinion of the day: after all, women belonged to the "domestic sphere" of life, and war was not a part of that sphere.[22] In order to be taken seriously, the WCAR had to become the United States Sanitary Commission, and needed to be run by men. President Lincoln signed it into official existence on June 13, 1861. Once the private relief agency was formed, supporting sick and wounded Union soldiers by collecting supplies and money became its primary mission. It was modeled after the British Sanitary Commission set up during the Crimean War and from the British parliamentary report published after the Indian Rebellion of 1857.[23]

Besides architect Frederick Law Olmstead, there were five other Sanitary Commissioners: Reverend Henry Whitney Bellows, George Templeton Strong, William H. Van Buren, M.D., Cornelius R. Agnew, and Professor Wolcott Gibbs, M.D. These men arrived in Washington almost immediately to meet with then-Secretary of War Simon Cameron for a tour of Union hospitals. Appalled by what they saw, these men—a unique combination of doctors, lawyers and politicians—soon began to organize a network that would eventually consist of approximately 7,000 soldiers' aid societies across the North and Midwest.[24]

These aid societies were mainly run by women and reached into the most humble households as well as the richest estates. Local groups of caring Northern women agreed to sew necessary articles in their homes and bring them (or have them picked up) to a central receiving area. From there, articles were collected into much larger packages of like items, and sent to regional depots. At the receiving points everything was sorted, inspected, packed, and sent to Union hospitals and camps. The branch women were so

21 Jeanie Attie, *Patriotic Toil: Northern Women and the American Civil War Publisher* (Ithaca: Cornell University Press, 1998), 53.

22 Nancy Woloch, *Women and the American Experience* (New York: McGraw Hill, 2006), 118.

23 United States Sanitary Commission Records, 1861-1872, New York Public Library, http://digitalgallery.nypl.org/nypldigital/id?1947303.

24 Judith Ann Geisburg, *Civil War Sisterhood: The U.S. Sanitary Commission and Women's Politics in Transition* (Boston: Northeastern University Press, 2000), 5.

successful in reaching out to faraway contributors that even the Pacific Coast donated approximately $1.5 million dollars as well as sewn or crafted items to Civil War relief.[25]

As the war progressed, the USSC volunteers created what were called Sanitary Fairs as a way to continue to raise money and encourage morale and support for Union soldiers. These enormous fairs provided exhibits featuring locally made items and were sponsored by local organizations. Another feature of the fairs was the travelling exhibits put together by USSC members living near Washington or close to battlegrounds. They collected "artifacts" and put together travelling exhibitions that were displayed prominently to the public. One popular exhibit was the uniform jacket worn by Colonel Elmer Ellsworth, shown along with the flag he captured from the Marshall House Hotel and a bayonet-adorned rifle claiming to have taken the life of hotel manager James Jackson. Entertainment and food were provided—all for a donation, of course. Commissioners travelled across the North to meet and negotiate with civic and business leaders, organize the construction of temporary buildings if necessary, and planning what would be offered at each individual fair. These endeavors raised nearly $3 million dollars (over 60 million dollars in today's currency) for branch treasuries, which helped them continue to supply donations for the Sanitary Commission.[26] The USSC leadership sometimes did not approve of the excitement and lavishness of the fairs. They wanted to encourage sacrifice as a component of membership. Although the fairs were one way to create a national identity that might motivate citizens to perform their duties, the men of the commission did not want the fairs to become the focus of USSC work.

Still, all that money was put to excellent use, with nary a whiff of corruption. The USSC provided for hospitals and camp clinics, and one of its first endeavors to get the sick and wounded away from the field of battle was to organize a group of hospital ships. In the spring of 1862, in coordination with Gen. McClellan's failed Seven Days' Battle on the Virginia Peninsula, hospital ships began to ferry wounded men from White House landing in Virginia, to Washington City. The doctors and nurses on board were overwhelmed with sick and dying soldiers. During one three-day period, they cared for approximately 2,000 men. Nurse Harriet Whetton wrote about

25 Attie, *Patriotic Toil*, 117.

26 Ibid., 3 and http://www.measuringworth.com.uscompare/.

the Union soldiers, held prisoner by the Confederacy for several days, who arrived on troop trains for passage aboard the hospital ships. "At first sight of the old Flag the poor boys set up a weak cheer and were so eager that they began to tumble and hobble out almost before the train stopped. They were in a wretched condition, their wounds full of maggots, their clothes full of vermin and nearly starved."[27] The newly commissioned USSC fleet, cobbled together from just about any floatable boat that could be rented or bought, got the men to hospitals.

As the war continued, the USSC became one of the most reliable sources for supplies necessary to the soldiers not yet provided by the government. Most of these supplies were used in Union hospitals, and included tables for writing in bed, wire cradles for the protection of wounded limbs, hospital gowns, water appliances for the wetting of applied bandages, books, checkerboards and dominoes, and tons of clothing and bedding to replace what was ruined by injury and illness.[28]

In addition to setting up and staffing hospitals, the USSC operated 30 soldiers' homes, lodges, or rest houses for traveling or disabled Union soldiers. Most of these closed shortly after the war, but Appomattox did not end USSC efforts. [29] Throughout the next two years, USSC commissioners and volunteers continued to work with Union veterans to secure their bounties, back pay, and help them apply for pensions. It supported the "health and hygiene" of all veterans, and oversaw the immediate home care of those who were returning as disabled veterans. They had a Department of General Relief that accepted donations for former soldiers, too.[30] After turning over most of its responsibilities to federal, state, and private agencies, the United States Sanitary Commission was finally disbanded in May 1866.[31]

27 Paul Hass, "A Volunteer Nurse in the Civil War: The Diary of Harriet Douglas Whetton," in *Wisconsin Magazine of History*, V, 49 (Spring 1965), 211.

28 *New York Times*, "Necessity of Sanitary Organization," Sunday, June 9, 1861.

29 The Sanitary Commission Bulletin, "Soldiers' Homes and Lodges" 3:1279.

30 Sanitary Commission, 14–15. Additionally, money donations were requested by the Sanitary Commission to support these military Union hospitals. George T. Strong, Treasurer of the Commission, 68 Wall Street, N.Y., and George S. Coe, Treasurer of Central Executive Committee, American Exchange Bank, N.Y., received these funds.

31 Ibid.

When Dr. Benton added the addendum to the letter he wrote to his parents on June 5, 1864, he was not exaggerating:

"I can cheerfully say for the Sanitary Commission that it is saving thousands and thousands of lives. J.D.B." A pretty good endorsement of something that was initially the idea of "intrusive women."[32]

by Meg Groeling

author of *The Aftermath of Battle:*
The Burial of the Civil War Dead (Savas Beatie, 2015)

32   Benton letter, quoted on page 62.

Appendix C

The Development of the Ambulance Corps

Basic human decency and compassion demand the prompt removal of maimed and wounded soldiers from the field of battle, if only to mitigate their pain and suffering. While such concerns may not be at the forefront in the minds of commanders, cogent military reasons exist to support such policies:

1. Lacking a systematic plan for the care and evacuation of the wounded, fighters tend to drop out of the ranks to assist fallen comrades, attenuating the strength of an attacking force.

2. Besides offering an outlet for the noble expression of human sympathy, casualties left on the field can also provide an excuse for faint-hearted men to shirk dangerous combat responsibilities, under the pretext of helping others make their way to the rear.

3. On the positive side, there is evidence that knowing trained and able men are waiting to assist those who fall, bolsters the morale and courage of troops under fire.

An organized ambulance corps did not exist at the beginning of the Civil War, but the need for such a service was clear to medical officers. In April 1862, Army of the Potomac Medical Director Charles S. Tripler called for the assignment of an experienced quartermaster and assistant commissary of subsistence to the command of the Chief Medical Officer of an army in the field. The duties of this office would include the acquisition, preparation, and operation of ambulance wagons, boats and hospital buildings.

Four months later, Surgeon General William A. Hammond submitted a proposal to Secretary of War Edwin M. Stanton, urging the creation of a Hospital Corps. "In no battle yet have the wounded been properly looked after; men under pretense of carrying them off the field leave the ranks and seldom return to their proper duties. The adoption of this plan would do away with the necessity of taking men from the line of the army to perform the duties of nurses, cooks, and attendants, and thus return sixteen thousand men to duty in the ranks."

General-in-Chief Henry W. Halleck vetoed the plan, citing the inevitable enormous costs, the enlargement of already too-long wagon trains, and a concern that "the presence of non-combatants on, or near the field of battle, is always detrimental, as most panics and stampedes originate with them."

Despite high-level objections to the formation of an army-wide Hospital Corps, Maj. Gen. McClellan issued General Orders No. 147 on August 2, 1862, for the creation of an Ambulance Corps within each of the army corps under his command. Those regulations called for the designation of a captain as commandant of each ambulance corps. He would command all ambulances and transport carts in his corps, under the supervision of the Medical Director of the Army of the Potomac, Surgeon Jonathan Letterman.

McClellan's orders established an organizational structure within each Ambulance Corps. A 1st lieutenant, acting as assistant quartermaster for the division ambulance corps, would have complete control of all ambulances, transport carts and ambulance horses within his division, as well as a travelling cavalry forge, a blacksmith, and a saddler to assist him in keeping his train in order. A 2nd lieutenant would command the ambulances of each brigade. A sergeant was to oversee the ambulances of each regiment, conducting necessary drills and inspections. The regulations specified that officers and non-commissioned officers of the ambulance details should be mounted.

Before any engagement, the captain received orders from the Medical Director concerning the distribution of ambulances and the points to which the wounded should be carried from the field. Light, two-horse ambulances transported casualties to a field station for preliminary evaluation and treatment, after which four-horse ambulances would convey patients farther to the rear for more definitive care.

The orders specified that corps commanders should select their ambulance details with great care, choosing only active and efficient men. Furthermore, only orders from Headquarters could relieve a man from this duty.

Two medical officers from the reserve corps of surgeons of each division, and a hospital steward assigned to the medicine wagon, accompanied the ambulance train when on the march. A member of the ambulance corps could treat and evacuate only wounded or sick persons belonging to his own corps.

The advantages of this organization were evident at the battle of Antietam in September 1862. By the night of September 18, just one day after the close of the battle, corpsmen had successfully completed the removal of all casualties to places of shelter and necessary medical attention. Contrary to Gen. Halleck's prediction, no panics or stampedes occurred among them. The triage system worked flawlessly. The results were equally favorable at Fredericksburg.

In the Army of the Tennessee, General Grant issued orders for the regulation of ambulance trains in March 1863.

In the spring of 1864, Congress passed, President Lincoln approved, and the Secretary of War promulgated through General Orders No. 106, an act that established a uniform ambulance system throughout the armies of the United States. This act consolidated authority over the Ambulance Corps within the Medical Department. Medical officers proved themselves worthy of the trust placed in them, by the systematic efficiency with which they handled the immense number of casualties that soon flowed from the battles of the Wilderness, Spotsylvania Courthouse, Cold Harbor, and Petersburg.

Transportation of the Wounded

Litters

Makeshift modes of conveying the wounded from the battlefield included the use of stout sticks or muskets passed through sleeves of a coat, or rolled into the edges of blankets, to form a primitive litter. Gates or ladders covered with blankets or straw made suitable stretchers in a pinch. Poles interlaced with ruptured telegraph wire could serve the same purpose.

In most cases, however, manufactured hand litters were used to accomplish the initial removal of wounded soldiers from the battlefield. The records of the property division of the Surgeon General's office show that the U. S. Army purchased and issued 52,489 litters of various types during the Civil War.

In the beginning of the war, the Satterlee ("U. S. Regulation") litter was the most common type. It weighed 24.5 pounds and was 27 inches wide. Two seasoned ash poles 1-1/2 inches in diameter and 8 feet 9 inches long, passed through 7-1/2-inch-wide pockets on either side of a canvas sling 5 feet 10 inches in length. Ropes attached to cross bars at either end stretched the canvas lengthwise. Adjustable leather shoulder straps, 2 inches wide, attached to the handles of the stretcher.

In 1862, Asst. Surgeon Henry S. Schell proposed a multipurpose litter that served as both a stretcher and bedstead. Strong hinges attached ten-inch handles to both ends of the 6 foot 2 inch parallel sidebars. In order to configure the litter as a cot in the hospital tent, the handles folded downward at right angles to form legs.

A great variety of other hand litters, litter carriages, and cacolets (seats or beds fitted to a mule to carry the sick or injured) appeared during the course of the war, but in general, those with an elegantly simple design proved most useful.

Ambulance Wagons

The armies of the United States did not use wagons designed specifically for the transport of wounded soldiers until shortly before the outbreak of the Civil War. Various designs were proposed, some of which were intricately complex, including tents that unfurled from the rooftops, and canvas slings that hung from the tops. Designers made continuous efforts to provide flexibility in bed and seating arrangements, and to improve the suspension, with the goal of providing increased levels of comfort for the human cargo.

In 1859, a board of medical officers recommended setting ambulance capacity at a ratio of 40 spaces per thousand soldiers. The board considered the two-wheel ambulance as the most convenient for transporting dangerously sick or wounded men, and a number of these carts saw service in the early part of the war. Experience soon proved them useless, however, as their motion was intolerable, prompting most occupants to beg for other options. Four-wheel vehicles, the earliest of which was the Tripler ambulance wagon (1859), supplanted them.

The spring-suspension Wheeling or Rosecrans ambulance wagon saw heavy service in the early part of the war. It was lighter than the Tripler, so that two horses could pull it, instead of the usual four. By adjusting the interior bench seating options, it could accommodate a dozen sitting patients, two recumbent and two or three sitting patients, or four recumbent patients. Fully accessorized, it included storage for stretchers, water tanks and a medicine box, a canvas cover and side curtains to protect against inclement weather, and a step at the rear to assist carriers in lifting in the wounded.

Brig. Gen. Daniel H. Rucker designed the preferred ambulance for latter part of the war. With a four-bed capacity, it had hinged stretchers that could also serve as seats. Lattice openings ventilated a 21-inch-deep space between the lower and upper levels of stretchers. The body of the wagon rested on platform springs, and the front wheels were smaller than those to the rear.

Mass Transportation

Commanders soon learned that rapid dispersion of the disabled was the most effective means of preserving the fighting force. Benefits of this strategy included: reduction of the need for combatants to leave their combat duties to assist sick and wounded comrades; elimination of the need for large accumulations of medical and hospital supplies in the field; lesser requirements for division, brigade, and regimental medical officers and hospital attendants to detach from marching columns (which typically already lacked adequate supplies and surgical expertise to deal with medical contingencies in the field).

The Union system of railroads and steamers greatly facilitated the speedy removal of sick and wounded soldiers from the scene of active operations, saving lives, alleviating suffering, and uncomplicating the prosecution of the war. After the battle of Gettysburg, 23,342 casualties came under the care of medical officers of the Army of the Potomac. Within two weeks, 15,425 had been forwarded to Baltimore, York, Harrisburg, and New York City. The efficiency of this evacuation improved after the battles of the Wilderness and Spotsylvania. With few exceptions, the wounded found comfortable shelter in hospitals at Alexandria, Washington, Baltimore, Philadelphia, and New York within just a few days of their injuries.

Specially outfitted railroad cars and ships proved particularly well-suited for the task of comfortably and efficiently transporting wounded men over long distances. When the Army was massed before the entrenched line at Petersburg for nine months, the large Depot Field Hospital at City Point, at the junction of the James and Appomattox Rivers, was connected with the positions of the several Army corps by a railroad with multiple branches. Sick and wounded from division hospitals traveled to the depot in box cars that had carried forward supplies for the troops. They were then transferred to hospital steamers, or retained at City Point for treatment, at the discretion of the Medical Director for Transportation, Surgeon Edward B. Dalton.

The principal boats employed for this task in the eastern waters were the steamers *Empress, Imperial, Connecticut, State of Maine, Western Metropolis, De Molay, Spaulding, Baltic, Atlantic, JK Barnes, Commodore, Cosmopolitan, Knickerbocker, Elm City,* etc. The capacity of the *Connecticut* was 400 patients. She made 47 trips and conveyed 18,919 patients.

Entering the Modern Era

With the organization of hospital systems, including local and long-distance transportation networks, Civil War medicine made major strides in the development of what we in modern times refer to as military and civilian trauma networks. Many present-day concepts find their origins in forward-thinking strategists from the Medical Corps in the American War of the Rebellion.

Primary Source: *The Medical and Surgical History of the War of the Rebellion*, 6 vols (Washington, D.C.: GPO, 1875), vol. 2, Chapter XV.

by Dennis Rasbach, M.D.

author of *Chamberlain at Petersburg: His Supposed Charge from Fort Hell, his Near-Mortal Wound, and a Civil War Myth Reconsidered*

Appendix D

Amputations in the Civil War

If a soldier was unfortunate enough to come under a surgeon's knife during the American Civil War, there is a high likelihood he emerged with one or more of his limbs missing. Amputation was the signature operation of the Civil War surgeon. An estimated 30,000 legs and arms were dismembered by Union surgeons during the war, accounting for seventy-five percent of all operations performed. The numbers were probably quite similar on the Confederate side.

It has been suggested that injuries to the extremities were more common than other injuries. This seems counterintuitive, and probably represents an anomaly of reporting.

Aside from the occasional sharpshooter, who presumably would have been aiming for a lethal head or chest wound, aiming in the Civil War was far from precise. The pattern of wounds inflicted by general infantry and artillery units should have conformed to a relatively random pattern, in proportion to the body surface area exposed. With the legs representing 36%, and the arms 18% of body surface, extremity wounds would be expected to comprise about half of all injuries, many of those being "flesh wounds" not requiring amputation. Indeed, of the 89,528 cases of injuries to the lower extremities entered on the permanent registers of the Surgeon General's office, as reported in *The Medical and Surgical History of the War of the Rebellion*, 59,376 were soft tissue wounds and 30,152 involved fractures, a ratio of two to one in favor of the soft tissue injuries. Thus, serious, irreparable extremity injuries requiring amputation could have accounted for only a quarter of battlefield wounds.

The simple fact is that Civil War surgeons had little to offer in the way of treatment for other serious injuries. The War of the Rebellion was one of the last major military conflicts to be decided in the era prior to the advent of our modern understanding of antisepsis and anesthesia. Without the benefit of that knowledge, surgery as we know it was largely impossible.

Civil War surgeons, with blood splattered clothes and unwashed hands, were notoriously unhygienic. They would often explore a wound with their bare fingers. Surgical Instruments were never sterilized. Dropped instruments were typically rinsed in cool, often bloody water, and sponges or bandages were frequently reused from patient to patient after a brief rinsing in cool water. It would be two years after the war's end before Joseph Lister would begin publishing his six articles on the Germ Theory of Disease in the British medical journal *Lancet*.

The main anesthetic agents available to Civil War surgeons were chloroform and ether. A few drops of the anesthetic were dripped onto a cloth that was placed over the face of the patient. This produced an unawareness of pain, but left the patient agitated, moaning, crying and thrashing about, having to be held still by assistants so the surgeon could do his work. The "anesthetic" was stopped quickly to minimize toxicity, necessitating quick work by the surgeon before the effect wore off. The first use of nitrous oxide as an inhalational anesthetic agent would not come until 1868, and intravenous solutions would not be developed until 1881.

Ninety percent of penetrating abdominal wounds were ultimately fatal, as were nearly two of three penetrating wounds to the chest. Civil war soldiers with wounds to the head or thorax were considered unsalvageable, which placed them at the bottom of the triage list for surgical care.

Types of Amputations

Civil War military manuals distinguished two basic types of amputations: those performed in the contiguity of the extremity (meaning a separation of adjacent bones by disarticulation), which required only a knife to divide the ligaments; and those that required disruption of the continuity of the limb, demanding the use of a saw or bone pliers to divide one or more of the long bones.

Soft tissue cuts could be made entirely from the surface moving inward toward the center through successive layers until the bony structures were encountered, or the amputation could include a partial cutting outward on one side of the limb, leaving a flap of viable tissue to facilitate closure.

Amputation Instruments

The basic surgical instrumentation for an amputation included a tourniquet; one or more knives to sever the soft tissues, an amputation saw, bone cutting pliers, forceps or tweezers, and a hook or tenaculum to snag the retracted blood vessels for ligation, once they had been severed.

The Theater of Operations

Amputations were usually performed in the open air to take advantage of daylight, which provided illumination far superior to that of kerosene lanterns or candles. As a result, the spectacle was by no means private, and observers were not limited to those with medical training or interest.

Technique of Amputation

Before beginning the operation, all necessary instruments, dressings etc., were placed in order, and within easy reach of the surgeon. The patient was positioned recumbent on a table. The skin was shaved for several inches above and below the line of incision. If an anesthetic was to be used (usually chloroform), it was important to make sure that the patient was fully under its influence.

The extremity to be removed was extended beyond the edge of the table, supported by an assistant. The limb's chief artery was controlled either by application of direct pressure, or preferably by application of a tourniquet, which was not tightened until just before the incision was to be made.

To help minimize blood loss, the limb could be elevated and a constricting bandage applied, wrapping from the distal end toward the amputation site to exsanguinate the tissues just prior to the application of the tourniquet.

The surgeon typically stood on the right of the diseased limb so that his left hand could rest upon and command the part to be saved. An assistant, grasping the whole circumference of the skin a short distance above the level of amputation would steadily and evenly stretch the skin.

Incision of the Soft Parts

In the circular method of amputation, the soft tissue was incised circumferentially, layer by layer, moving from the skin toward the bone at the center. The operator, stooping and encircling the limb with his right arm, held the long amputating knife like a sword with its point aimed downward and toward himself, the heel of the instrument resting on the skin to be divided. The incision was continued with a gentle sawing motion drawing the blade completely around the circumference of the limb to the spot where the cut had commenced, the surgeon's hand beginning prone and extended, then supinating, and ending up prone and flexed. During the progress of the procedure the surgeon would rise from his stooped position, resuming an erect posture by the end of the maneuver. Some operators preferred to make two semicircular cuts, a technique that was equally efficient, but one that was somewhat lacking in showmanship and finesse.

The first incision was intended to divide the skin and subcutaneous tissue down to the deep fascial layer investing the muscle. The cut was made perpendicular to the skin surface. The first cut was followed by two subsequent incisions in the muscle layers, each one made in line with the margin of the overlying structures that were being strongly retracted proximally by the assistant. The effect of retracting the overlying tissues during the successive cuts resulted in a hollow conoidal wound, the apex of which was the bone, which was then divided with a saw.

An alternate approach was to amputate by the creation of flaps. Any proportion between the flaps could be obtained as required by the individual case. To secure a good stump, it was necessary to increase the length of one flap in the same portion that the other was reduced.

Sectioning the Bone

Using a hand saw, the division of the bone was begun on a horizontal axis, shifting to an oblique angle and then finishing the cut with the saw vertical and moving toward the surgeon.

Ligation of the Vessels

As a general rule, only the arteries needed to be secured with ligatures. Lower pressure venous bleeding was controlled by elevation of the stump, and only when bleeding persisted was the vein tied off.

Dressings

Once all bleeding was controlled, the raw wound surface was cleansed with cold water and a sponge. Skin edges were brought into as near-perfect apposition as possible with sutures, adhesive strips or bandages, leaving some opening through which pus could drain. Available suture materials may have included horsehair, waxed silk, cotton or flax thread, or metallic wire.

Outcomes

Of the nearly 55,000 Civil War amputations officially reported on both sides of the conflict, the estimated overall mortality was 30 percent. Mortality was higher, the more proximal the level of amputation, ranging from 6 percent at the foot or toe, to 25 percent at the ankle joint, to 58 percent at the knee joint, and 83 percent at the hip. Amputations performed before the onset of shock (within the first hour) had the best results. When performed between the first and sixth hour after injury, results were somewhat less successful, but better than those that were done later. The poorest results occurred with surgery between the forty-eighth hour and the seventh day.

Modern Progress?

Techniques of amputation have, in some respects, changed very little over the past 150 years. The procedure still involves the incision of soft tissues, which is now most commonly done with a scalpel and by creating flaps, rather than with the circular technique that was so popular in the Civil War. The bone can be divided with electrical or battery-operated mechanical oscillating saws, although many times it is still cut with a hand saw or a Gigli two-handed wire saw. The long amputation knife is still in the equipment set, as are pliers-like bone cutters and a bone file that looks very much like a carpenter's rasp.

What has changed radically is the availability of safe general anesthesia. Surgeons are no longer under constraints to work rapidly before the anesthetic wears off, or becomes lethal. Instead of taking ten minutes, as was typical in the Civil War era, a modern amputation may consume nearly an hour. The procedure is performed in an operating room, with intense artificial illumination, under very controlled circumstances, using strict sterile technique.

The indications for amputation have shifted over time, along with changes in longevity and lifestyle. In a twenty-first century civilian surgical practice, infection and gangrene from poor circulation have replaced traumatic injury as the main reason for amputation. Instead of operating on healthy young adult men, modern surgeons typically operate on middle-aged or elderly individuals with peripheral vascular disease and diabetes, often associated with renal failure requiring dialysis. Tourniquets are rarely used in these circumstances, out of concern for potential compromise of the tenuous blood supply, which would adversely affect the viability of the amputation stump. In this frail population, the early mortality is not much better than it was in the pre-antibiotic, pre-anesthetic Civil War population, with 22 percent of lower extremity amputees not surviving 30 days. Unfortunately, that is not the end of the story. In the setting of chronic diabetes, renal failure, and cardiovascular disease, 44 percent of amputees will be dead by one year; and 77 percent will have succumbed by five years after the surgery.

Select Bibliography

Barnes, J. K. (1876). *Medical and Surgical History of the War of the Rebellion, Surgical History*, Part 2, Vol. 2. Washington: Government Printing Office.

Bollet, A. J. "The Truth about Civil War Surgery," in *Civil War Times* (June 2006), www.historynet.com/the-truth-about-civil-war-surgery-2.htm (accessed February 19, 2017).

Fortington, L. V. "Short and Long Term Mortality Rates after a Lower Limb Amputation," in *European Journal of Vascular and Endovascular Surgery* (July 2013), 46 (1), 124- 131.

Gross, S. D. *A Manual of Military Surgery* (Philadelphia: J. B. Lippincott, 1862).

"Maimed Men. Retrieved from Life and Limb: The Toll of the American Civil War." www.nlm.nih.gov/exhibition/lifeandlimb/maimedmen.html.

Civil War Battlefield Surgery. Retrieved from ehistory: https://ehistory.osu.edu/ exhibitions/ cwsurgeon/cwsurgeon/amputations.

Rutkow, I. M. Chapter 5, "Civil War Surgery," in *Surgery: An Illustrated History*. 1861-1865 (Philadelphia: Lippincott-Raven, 1993).

by Dennis Rasbach, M.D.

author of *Chamberlain at Petersburg: His Supposed Charge from Fort Hell, his Near-Mortal Wound, and a Civil War Myth Reconsidered*

Appendix E

Civil War Dressings—Lint

In reading Dr. Benton's correspondence, most of the medical terminology was familiar to me as a practicing surgeon. However, one statement from the Introduction caught my attention:

> A typical regimental knapsack would contain both chloroform and ether for use as anesthetics, lint, bandages, tourniquets, sponges, morphine, opium pills, whiskey, and brandy. . . . After foreign particles were removed, the wound would then be packed with lint, bandaged, and the soldier would be directed toward the ambulance collecting point where he would be picked up and transported to a field hospital farther to the rear.

What was the significance of lint in Civil War medicine? How was it procured in quantity for use by military surgeons? And how, exactly, was it employed in the treatment of battlefield wounds? My curiosity was piqued!

The short answer is that lint was a fluffy absorbent material, made from linen cloth, that was applied to open wounds to help control bleeding and to wick away excess moisture and drainage—probably an antiquated precursor to our modern calcium alginate, or Kaltostat. It was manufactured, to some extent, in the North, but was also manually produced on a massive scale, in both the North and South, by women and children doing their part for the war effort by working in small groups at home, or at ladies' relief societies. However, there is much more to the story. As it so happens, the fiber that we would simply discard as waste from our modern electric clothes dryers turns out to be an essential element in the successful treatment of battlefield injuries during the Civil War and beyond.

The best available primary source for a detailed description of the medical applications of lint is Henry Hollingsworth Smith's 1850 textbook *Minor Surgery; or, Hints on the Every-Day Duties of the Surgeon*. Smith begins this more-than-three-hundred-page treatise with a highly technical discussion of the preparation and application of surgical dressings:

> The Pieces of Dressing are Lint; Charpie; Cotton; Tow; Spread Cerate, or other ointment; Compresses; Maltese Cross; Shields for Amputations; Adhesive Strips; Setons; Poultices; Plasters; and Irrigations.

> Lint is a soft, delicate tissue or mass, prepared in two ways;—in one of which the transverse threads of soft old linen are drawn out by a machine, leaving the longitudinal ones covered by a sort of tomentum or cotton-like mass; the other, in which the cotton-like surface is produced by scraping, with a sharp knife, a similar piece of cloth, previously fastened to some firm substance. The first is known as the Patent Lint, and may be obtained at any apothecaries, as it is now generally manufactured; the second, is the Domestic Lint, and may be made at a moment's notice where the first is not convenient. They are both employed as primary dressings, either spread with ointments or alone.

Henry Smith then embarks on a lengthy description of charpie, another form of lint:

> Charpie is a substance much employed by the French surgeons, and worthy of a more general application in the United States. It consists of a collection of filaments, separated from morsels of old linen rag, four or five inches square, of loose texture, and well calculated to absorb. It is divided into two kinds, according to the length and fineness of the thread composing it; that which is long and coarse being employed to keep open sinuses, fistulas, and as an outer dressing, while the softer, finer kind may be placed in immediate contact with the part, especially where the surface requires stimulation.

Various names were assigned to charpie, according to the way in which its fibers were arranged before its application. There was the Plumasseau,

Bourdonnet, Tente, Mèche, Boulette, Tampon, and Pelote; each of which had its particular advantages.

Plumasseau

Plumasseau was a mass of parallel charpie filaments, the ends of which were folded under and flattened between the palms of the hands. The result was a thick mass with rounded edges, which the physician then coated with "cerate," an unctuous preparation consisting of wax or resin mixed with oil, lard and medicinal ingredients. Smith's treatise warns that care should be taken not to make the Plumasseau "so thick as to overload and heat the part, nor yet so thin as to become quickly saturated with the pus."

Bourdonnet

The Bourdonnet was a smaller mass of charpie, made by rolling linen fibres between the hands to create an oblong cylinder that was tied in the middle and then folded in half, forming a cone-shaped plug. This was used for absorbing pus in deep-seated wounds that had a tendency to close at the surface before the bottom had filled in. It was also used to stop bleeding from vessels deep within the soft tissues, the thick central core serving to compress the vessel, and the more loosely dispersed end fibers facilitating formation of a clot.

Tente

The Tente was a conical mass of charpie, similar to the Bourdonnet, except there was no string tied around its middle. Instead, after folding it in half, the loose ends were twisted, giving it a spiral shape. It was used to dilate fistulous channels that were too small to allow of the free escape of pus.

Sponge Tente

In situations where the walls of a sinus tract were rigid, the Sponge Tente was preferred. This was made by slicing gentian, carrot, or some other porous root, or by saturating common sponge with melted bees-wax, allowing it to cool and harden, and then slicing it into small pieces that would nearly fill the tract to be dilated. Body heat would melt the wax, allowing the sponge to absorb exudate generated by the wound, dilating and maintaining the orifice in the process.

Boulettes

Boulettes were little balls of different sizes, made by rolling charpie between the hands. Porous and absorbent, they were used to fill and distend cavities of pus, or to arrest bleeding. When multiple Boulettes were packed together at the bottom of a cavity, they were said to form a Tampon. Such an application was often employed (off the battlefield) in the treatment of vaginal gonorrhea and to arrest uterine hemorrhage. Boletus lgniarius, the puff-ball of botany, was also employed for these purposes.

Pelote

The Pelote was a large boulette, surrounded by a piece of soft rag, the edges of which are brought together and tied firmly. It was used as a truss in the treatment of hernia, but also in the compression of large vessels, such as the axillary artery, and to control hemorrhage from the rectum.

Cotton and Maggots

Lint was similar in some respects to cotton, but cotton was inferior for most medical purposes, other than as a dressing for burns. Civil War surgeons chose cotton for use in burn patients to protect the denuded surface from the air and to absorb the discharge, forming a sort of scab under which the burn would heal. However, the use of cotton was associated with the unwanted generation of maggots:

> When intended to be thus used, it is especially necessary to see that it is free even from specks, as the fly is exceedingly apt to lay its egg here, where it is vivified by the heat of the body, and generates maggots, to the great annoyance of the patient and the astonishment of all around him, as they are unable to account for their appearance, and regard it as a fatal sign.

Interestingly, the lowly fly larva has benefited from a modern-day make over of its image within the medical community. Disinfected "germ-free" medical maggots are now available by prescription for the debridement of open wounds. According to the supplier, proteolytic enzymes dissolve dead and infected tissue; antimicrobial secretions disinfect the wound and dissolve biofilm; maggots ingest and kill microbes within their guts; and their presence in the wound stimulates the growth of healthy tissue!

Production of Lint during the Civil War

Both patent (machine produced) and domestic scraped lint were essential medical supplies for the armies of the North and South during the Civil War. U. S. Army regulations specified that four pounds of patent lint and two pounds of scraped lint should be stocked in a properly-equipped medical wagon, and a half pound of patent lint was needed for a medical pannier. The Confederate army regulations recommended eight pounds for a regiment, four pounds for a battalion, and two pounds for a company for three months. Of course, the necessary amounts would vary with the battle experience of any given unit, and as the fighting intensified, it became evident that these recommended quantities of lint would be woefully inadequate.

Soon after the beginning of the war, Southern newspapers began to publicize the impending need for this scarce commodity. On April 26, 1861, a writer in the Natchez Daily Courier appealed to the patriotism of the women of that city and county to furnish the military stores with charpie "prepared out of old worn-out shirts and sheets, which are commonly thrown away. 'Save the pieces;' cut them in squares of 4 or 5 inches, pick them, and the required article is prepared. If it is sweet to bleed for the country, it is not less sweet to know that the wounds will be dressed properly; moreover, by the handwork of our mothers and sisters."

Diaries, letters and memoirs of the period contain many references to the preparation of lint by ladies' relief societies on both sides of the Mason Dixon Line. The fact that the Confederacy did not have a source of manufactured lint available throughout the war, made the need for home production especially acute in the South.

According to the *Medical and Surgical History of the War of the Rebellion*, 147,135 pounds of patent lint, and 82,754 pounds of scraped or picked linen were purchased or manufactured in the North during the Civil War. It is unclear whether these totals include the hundreds of pounds of lint shipped by the relief organizations, such as the Sanitary Commission, to northern hospitals.

Lint was an essential element in the treatment of battlefield injuries during the Civil War. Surgeons continued to use both lint and charpie until sterile gauze pads were introduced, just before World War I.

Select Bibliography

Mescher, Virginia. "Lint and Charpie: It's Not Your Dryer Lint" (2003). See www.raggedsoldier.com/lint.pdf.

Smith, Henry H. Minor Surgery; or, Hints on the Every-Day Duties of the Surgeon. Philadelphia: E. Barrington & G. D. Haswell, 1850.

by Dennis Rasbach, M.D.

author of *Chamberlain at Petersburg: His Supposed Charge from Fort Hell, his Near-Mortal Wound, and a Civil War Myth Reconsidered*

Sources

Published Books

Adams, George W. *Doctors in Blue: The Medical History of the Union Army in the Civil War, 5th edition*. Louisiana State University Press: Baton Rouge, LA, 1996.

Adams, George W. "Caring for the Men," in William C. Davis and Bill I. Wiley, eds., Civil War Album: Complete Photographic History of the Civil War Fort Sumter to Appomattox. Tess Press: New York, NY, 2000.

Billings, John D. *Hard Tack and Coffee: Soldier's Life in the Civil War*. Konecky & Konecky: 2004.

Biographical Review: The Leading Citizens of Cayuga County New York. Biographical Review Publishing Company: Boston, MA, 1894.

Bowen, John. *Battlefields of the Civil War: A State by State Guide. Chartwell Books Inc: NJ, 1986.*

Catton, Bruce. *The Civil War*. Houghton Mifflin Company: Boston, MA, 1988.

Cecil, Russell L, and Foster Kennedy, eds., *A Text Book of Medicine by American Authors. W.B. Saunders Company: Philadelphia, PA, 1928.*

Coco, Gregory A. A *Strange and Blighted Land: Gettysburg The Aftermath of a Battle*. Thomas Publications: Gettysburg, PA, 1995.

——. *A Vast Sea of Misery: A History and Guide to the Union and Confederate Field Hospitals at Gettysburg July 1-November 20, 1863. Thomas Publications, Gettysburg, PA, 1988.*

———. *The Civil War Infantryman: In Camp, on the March, and in Battle.* Thomas Publications, Gettysburg, PA, 1996.

Confederate States Medical and Surgical Journal. Ayres & Wade: Richmond, VA, 1864.

Donald, David H. ed., *Gone for a Soldier: The Civil War Memoirs of Private Alfred Bellard. Little Brown and Company: Boston, MA, 1991.*

Dyer, Frederick H. *Compendium of the War of The Rebellion, 3 vols.* The Dyer Publishing Company: Des Moines, IA, 1908.

Freeman, Frank R. *Gangrene and Glory: Medical Care During the American Civil War.* University of Illinois Press: Chicago, IL, 2001.

Harwell, Richard. *Lee, An Abridgement in One Volume of the Four-Volume R.E. Lee by Douglas Southall Freeman.* New York: Simon & Schuster, 1997.

Husk, Martin W. *The 111th New York Volunteer Infantry: A Civil War History.* McFarland & Co: Jefferson, NC, 2010.

Kauffman, Michael W. *American Brutus: John Wilkes Booth and the Lincoln Conspiracies. Random House: New York, 2004.*

McHugh, Michael J. *George B. McClellan: The Disposable Patriot. Christian Liberty Press: Arlington Heights, IL, 1998.*

Miller, Frank, H Lyons Hunt, F. J McCormick, Morris King, and Buchanan Burr, eds., *Domestic Medical Practice: A Household Advisor in the Treatment of Diseases, Arranged for Family Use.* Chicago: Domestic Medical Society, 1926.

Murfin, James V. *Battlefields of the Civil War.* CLB Publishing: CT, 1990.

Pfanz, Donald C. *War So Terrible: A Popular History of the Battle of Fredericksburg. Page One History Publications: Richmond, VA, 2003.*

Phisterer, Frederick. New York in the War of the Rebellion, 6 vols. J.B. Lyon Company State Printers: Albany, NY, 1912.

Record of the Commissioned Officers, Non-Commissioned Officers and Privates of the Regiments Which Were Organized in the State of New York, vol. II. Comstock and Cassidy Printers: Albany, NY, 1864.

Robertson Jr., James I. *The Medical and Surgical History of the War of the Rebellion,* 6 Vols. Broadfoot Publishing Company: Wilmington, NC, 1991.

Sheldon, George. *When the Smoke Cleared at Gettysburg: The Tragic Aftermath of the Bloodiest Battle of the Civil War. Cumberland House: Nashville, TN, 2003.*

Smith, Edward P. *Incidents of the U.S. Christian Commission.* RJMC Publications: Concord, VA, 2003.

Sommers, Richard J. *Richmond Redeemed: The Siege of Petersburg.* Doubleday and Company Inc: Garden City, NJ, 1981.

Speer, Lonnie R. *Portals to Hell: Military Prisons of the Civil War.* Stackpole Books: Mechanicsburg, PA, 1997.

Storke, Elliot G. *History of Cayuga County, New York.* Heart of the Lakes Publishing: NY, 1980.

Tagg, Larry. *The Generals of Gettysburg: The Leaders of America's Greatest Battle.* Da Capo Press: MA, 1998.

Thomas, Dean S. *Ready, Aim, Fire: Small Arms Ammunition in the Battle of Gettysburg.* Thomas Publications: Gettysburg, PA, 1993.

Warner, Ezra J. *Generals in Blue.* LSU Press: Baton Rouge, LA, 1964.

Willey, Henry. *Isaac Willey of New London Connecticut and His Descendants.* E. Anthony and Sons Printers: New Bedford, MA, 1888.

Woodworth, Steven E and Kenneth J. Winkle. *Atlas of the Civil War.* Oxford University Press: New York, 2014.

Magazine Article

Campbell, Eric. "Remember Harper's Ferry: The Degradation, Humiliation, and Redemption of Col. George L. Willard's Brigade," in *Gettysburg Magazine.* July 1992. Issue 7, Part 1.

Newspapers

Gugliotta, Guy. "New Estimate Raises Civil War Death Toll," in New York Times. April 3, 2012. D1.

Internet Sources

American Chemical Society National Historic Chemical Landmarks. Development of the Pennsylvania Oil Industry. www.acs.org/content/acs/en/education/whatischemistry/landmarks/pennsylvaniaoilindustry.html, accessed on September 25, 2017.

William T. Sherman to James M. Calhoun, E.E. Rawson, and S.C. Wells, September 12, 1864. https://cwnc.omeka.chass.ncsu.edu/items/show/23, accessed on November 1, 2017.

Watkins, George H. http://files.usgwarchives.net/ga/military/civilwar/ rosters/12thbatt.txt. Web, last accessed on November 6, 2017.

Index

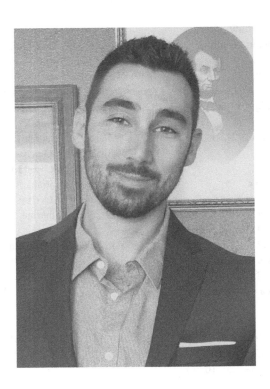

About the Author

Christopher E. Loperfido, a native of Weedsport, New York, graduated from Oswego State University with a bachelor's degree in history and political science. Chris worked for the National Park Service at Gettysburg National Military Park in the summers of 2007 and 2008 as both a park intern and National Park Service Ranger. He is currently employed by the Department of Homeland Security and lives with his wife, son, and pug in Washington State. *Death, Disease, and Life at War* is his first book.